Recipe for a Heart Attack
The Body's Perfect Storm

by

Elliot Brown, M.D., F.A.C.C.

DORRANCE PUBLISHING CO., INC.
PITTSBURGH, PENNSYLVANIA 15222

ISBN: 978-1-4349-0546-8
Printed in the United States of America

First Printing

For information or to order additional books, please write:
Dorrance Publishing Co., Inc.
701 Smithfield St.
Pittsburgh, Pennsylvania 15222
U.S.A.
1-800-788-7654
www.dorrancebookstore.com

Dedication

This book is dedicated to my wife, Maria, who has been an inspiration in my life, and as a cardiac cath lab nurse has helped me save countless lives; to my children, Russell, Leanne, Julie, and Jessica, who have taught me more about myself than they will ever know; to Dr. Stephen Dranoff, and to my very giving parents, Myrna and Jerry.

Contents

Introduction: Somewhere under the Radar

Throughout the course of my practice in adult cardiology and the study of humans, there have been many oxymorons that have plagued me. Why is it that a person can have a close brush with death, too close for comfort, in fact, and yet continue to smoke cigarettes? How do people find themselves greater than fifty pounds overweight in the doctor's office and insist they are following their diabetic diet? Why can't patients maintain a regular exercise program? The answers to these questions are very complex, and sometimes take a lifetime of work by the individual. Knowing the *right* thing to do isn't the problem. Patient education, while lacking to some extent in the average medical practice setting, is not the culprit. After all, America is not a nation deficient on the intellectual side of things. People are emotionally incapable of achieving the proper psychological health that is, in this physician's opinion, the key ingredient to obtaining and maintaining proper physical health and well being.

Thus, the gap between intellect and emotion forms the great human mystery to me as a practitioner. So much of the emotional "baggage" we bring to adulthood plays out in this gap. We know what we *should* do, but often choose what we *feel like* doing. It is the proverbial war between the body and the soul, between the child in us and the adult, etc. We struggle with it our entire lives. I have come to believe that our true work as humans during our time here on Earth is to do whatever it takes to best understand ourselves and why our own personal gap exists. To be or not to be. The result of this journey bridges the emotional and intellectual gap, and its ripple effect enables a meaningful life, complete with the wisdom necessary to give one clarity on what the *right* thing to do is and how to go about doing it.

I have seen the three hundred pound patient waddle into my office with the newest copy of "Reducing Cardiac Risk in 5 Easy Steps." Other than the exercise he gains from toting this overweight tome, I have never seen his health benefit from his library in the ten years I've known him. Yet he can quote some of the greatest nutrition gurus in the world. I have seen the patient who survived a premature myocardial infarction (MI, or heart attack) answer the question, "Why are you still smoking?" with a smile and a meek exclamation: "I heard there is some research data that shows that smoking reduces your risk of Alzheimer's disease!" Hello, sir, but even if that were true, perhaps it's because smokers don't live long enough to develop Alzheimer's disease!

There is no shortage of patients to use as examples when it comes to identifying who has a wide gap and how it manifests itself in his or her life. Many cases are not so obvious. There is the motivated young woman, college age or older, who has persistent palpitations that disable her. She has no demonstrable heart disease other than occasional benign skips on an electrocardiogram (EKG) recording. Nevertheless, her symptoms and subjective feelings of fear and doom are real. No matter how much you reassure the patient that she is okay, she continues to have an exaggerated interpretation of feelings of doom and symptoms of heart pounding. Sounds like intellectual and emotional mismatch, doesn't it? While it can manifest itself in different forms, this gap is as important to recognize as any other clinical finding is, or perhaps, as you will see, it is even more important.

Some patients demonstrate obvious emotional maladies. Depression and bipolar disorder (manic depression) are extremely common in and around a cardiology practice. There is increasingly emerging data linking depression, an affective disorder, to heart disease, and clinical trials are underway to determine if treatment of the depression with medication affects cardiovascular mortality. In addition to the affective disorders that have profound effects on cardiovascular outcomes, there are chronic stress disorders, such as job stress, marital stress, and caregiver stress, that have also been shown to play quite a significant role with respect to clinical cardiovascular outcomes. Animal models exist that link stress as a subjective emotional reaction that results in hormonal and physiological changes, which when present chronically result in worsened cardiovascular survival. Having established the physiological link of the mind-body interaction, behavioral cardiology is now a budding field pioneering this new frontier. Following the development of overt cardiac disease, anxiety disorders are quite prevalent, including post-traumatic stress disorder (PTSD) and panic attacks. By virtue of their activation of our unconscious nervous system, these emotional disorders also result in hormonal release that worsens cardiac prognosis over time.

Thus, we are living in a time when we know more than ever that there is a direct link between emotional status and heart disease. Psychosocial stress factors and depression have now been recognized as major risk factors and culprits in the etiology and progression of arteriosclerosis. Emotional factors such as depression and chronic stress lead to increases in circulating noradrenaline and cortisol levels. This in turn leads to increases in blood pressure and heart rate, and a tendency toward obesity and diabetes. Obesity, hypertension, and diabetes, when present together, comprise the "metabolic syndrome." People who have this syndrome represent the highest cardiovascular risk group on the planet. Many of these patients are in this condition because of their inability to follow the age-old axioms of regular exercise, weight loss, smoking cessation, limitation of alcohol and sodium, and avoidance of foods high in saturated fat or trans-fatty acids. There is nothing new about the above behavioral modification suggestions. Intellect is not the problem. There is also nothing new about our inability, as a culture, to follow these suggestions. What is new, therefore, is not the recognition and re-stating of the problem. It is the recognition that there is a common emotional denominator to it all. It is far below, in a place underneath the radar, that the real cure lies.

Realizing that many patients are often incapable of making the appropriate behavioral modifications is the keyhole to viewing the battleground. Why does one choose these intellectually *wrong* choices? These behaviors or gestures are nothing more than an emotionally adaptive response to something deep inside. Fear. Insecurity. Anxiety. Anger. Hostility. Sadness. Our population is so full of these emotions, yet in our lives, there is nowhere to put them. So, patients hide behind their behaviors, and *the behaviors* become the focus. Humans are wired to deceive themselves over and over again. Our society seeks pleasure, not healthy solutions to dealing with pain and difficulty. We live in a society of mania and fun, which gives us all the idea that problems are for the "other people." "Don't bother me; I'm having too good a time. By the way, do you have a pill for this?"

Realizing that you can't stop smoking after you've had your chest cracked open is obviously not enough. You are obligated to ask the tough questions, like "Why am I seeking emotional comfort this way knowing my behavior is going to kill me?" It is time to help patients open their Pandora's box. I am hopeful that this book will educate readers as to the mind-body nature of cardiovascular disease and make current concepts in the field truly tangible. But again, intellect isn't the problem. So, I am going to further develop for readers those common emotional themes people take into adulthood from their individual life experiences, and I hope they will recognize how these emotional factors have manifested themselves in their lives and how these factors are affecting their physical health. I aim to aid readers in identifying what is operative in their lives behind the many smokescreens of maladaptive behavior.

For the longest time my desire was to write the ultimate cardiology book for the patient, a book that teaches all one would want to learn about cardiac risk factors, hypertension, diabetes, smoking cessation, and the like. It would teach about medications and empower patients with some basic medical knowledge in order to arm them in their battles against atherosclerosis and cardiovascular disease. As I have said before, I have come to realize that the intellectual side of the disease is not the underlying problem. To truly have a profound effect on people's lives and help cure them of a disease, I have learned, you must be an expert at treating the physical malady, but you must also be an expert in "curing" patients from themselves. Such a cure lies somewhere below; somewhere under the radar.

So, how do you help the patients help themselves? I have long known that recognition of the problem is the first step toward improving it, and you must help patients recognize that the way they are living their lives is nothing more than a recipe brewing the perfect storm, resulting in a heart attack. The shelves are stocked with literature that wonderfully illustrates for the reader what to eat, how to cook it, when and how to exercise, how to relax, etc. While these sources are essential as part of the knowledge required to combat cardiovascular disease, America's number one killer of men and women, they don't necessarily help readers recognize that they themselves in fact contain the perfect storm in progress. These books leave room for the "This doesn't really apply to me" syndrome. But if you embody what this book is about, I hope that on a personal level you will come to realize that you are the one who needs to begin to make changes. A person cannot adopt a lifestyle change without truly knowing inside that he or she is headed down a frightful road.

*

Coincident with my journey into the human body and human nature, we will begin with cardiovascular disease, which is where it all started for me. Back in 1986, I was doing my psychiatric rotation in my third year of medical school at Lincoln Hospital in the Bronx. I had not yet rotated through medicine or surgery, and thus had not been exposed to many of the roles that major specialty groups fill within the practice of medicine. On this particular day, one of the patients attempted to commit suicide in her room on the inpatient psychiatric ward. When she was found by one of the nurses, a "code blue" was called. The next thing I knew, for the first time, I witnessed the "code team" come racing down the hall to our patient with "the paddles," the heart monitor, and the code cart, full of all types of syringes, medications, and resuscitation tools. There was one guy who had white pants on, and his stethoscope was draped around his neck like a necklace. He stood behind the EKG machine and barked out orders as he ran the code. I knew right then and there, that was the guy I wanted to be. I thought these types were the "warriors" of the medical staff. The goalies. When the puck got by everyone else, they had to stop it...or else. And, when the patient was resuscitated from a flat line, they got all the glory, as if they had scored the game winner in overtime.

I was convinced that to save lives, I had to go into internal medicine and, eventually, cardiology. What other discipline could give one such instant gratification? Suddenly, I wanted to know every detail about how the heart worked, and every detail about how to fix it. As far as I was concerned, this psychiatry stuff was interesting, but would only come in handy if I had a "crazy" patient sometime. Sitting around talking about feelings was not included in my definition of saving lives. Besides, when the patient needed resuscitation, the psychiatrists looked so uncomfortable taking care of the patient's medical condition; I actually questioned whether or not they were even included in my definition of what a doctor did at all!

So, it was off to St. Luke's Hospital in New York for three years of internal medicine residency and three more years of cardiology fellowship. It was a very exciting time in cardiology. In the mid and late 1980s we witnessed the revolution of thrombolytic therapy for acute myocardial infarction. In other words, we developed those "clot buster" medicines that for the first time could abort a heart attack while in progress and limit the amount of permanent injury to the heart muscle. This had been unheard of up until that point in time. We also perfected angioplasty with the use of balloons, rotational devices, plaque slicing devices, lasers, and most recently, metal and drug coated stents. Coronary bypass graft surgery was also advanced by the proficient use of the left internal mammary artery, and now surgery is routinely performed without shutting off the heart and putting it on a "cardiopulmonary bypass machine." The new method is called "off pump" surgery, which is safely done with and without mini incisions.

Yes, we certainly have become more and more effective at the acute treatment of coronary artery disease. We are great at taking the highest risk patients in the state of New Jersey and reducing them to low risk so they can begin to work on their risk factors and alter the outcome of their disease. In the overall treatment of coronary disease, I thought we had truly developed the cure, but in reality, I have come to realize that all we really do is buy some time to allow the patient to change things around for him or herself.

That's when it hit me. After years of feeling like I was among the lifesavers of the medical staff and "supreme warrior" in the trenches treating the most critically ill, I realized I was not saving anybody. I was just putting my finger in the dyke. Yes, after years of the patient fueling the plaque build-up, the fallacious notion was that the coronary disease was starting with me right then and there in the emergency room. "How could this be?...I was feeling perfect yesterday." The truth is, by the time the patient gets to me, there has already been a long, mature disease process going on in his or her coronary arteries for many years. The plaque is now ripe, and *boom*...MI. The fact is, the plaque that erupted on the day of the heart attack actually began to grow decades before.

Our ability to handle the acute presentations of coronary disease is, thankfully, quite good. In addition, over the course of practicing cardiology, the common regimen for the treatment of coronary disease has become: judicious treatment with beta-blockers, aggressive application of statins for cholesterol management, the application of platelet inhibitors such as aspirin and clopidogrel to thin the blood, and the additional use of ACE (angiotensin converting enzyme) inhibitors, and later ARBs (angiotensin receptor blockers). This "recipe" of drugs has become the mainstay of treatment, and has resulted in profound improvements in mortality rates and outcomes in the vast majority of patients. Our medical therapy is so good for the treatment and prevention of coronary disease that we are now reaching a plateau, or "maxing out," with respect to the effect we can have on coronary disease and our patients' outcomes.

For years I watched countless patients undergo coronary artery bypass graft surgery (CABG, pronounced "cabbage" surgery). I attended to people of all races, incomes, and sexes as they went through open-heart procedures. Many people were very successful at adopting a new lifestyle by taking on regular exercise, changing their diets, and stopping smoking. A significant portion of those people, however, after six months, a year, or maybe more, would revert back to a more sedentary lifestyle, old smoking habits, or uncontrolled weight gain, abandoning their "improved" healthy habits. Do patients really have such a poor memory? Do they really forget what has just happened to them? I suspect they feel so well again that they go back into their old "comfort zones" and lose the ability to stick to their newly adopted lifestyles.

Patients read all types of websites, books, and whatever they can get their hands on. Yet they smoke, they don't exercise, they eat too many fats and carbohydrates, and they fail to manage their diabetes and blood pressure aggressively. The mismatch between what they know and how they behave is what I refer to as "intellectual-emotional" mismatch.

Once the medical management of the disease became relatively standard, the psychological aspect of my patients became the most fascinating. If only I could help my patients learn what was inhibiting them from treating themselves better, I would really be able to have an effect on their illness and begin to heal them. I also recognized that the average patient with coronary disease has an internist and a cardiologist, goes to cardiac rehabilitation, may have a diabetes doctor, a urologist, etc., and is therefore unlikely to want to begin to see a psychologist to figure all of this out when simply referred. The patient already goes to enough appointments!

As the treating physician, it became incumbent upon me to explore the intellectual-emotional mismatch within my patients without referring each one to yet another specialist. The patient is a captive audience for the cardiologist. The experience of cardiac catheterization, coronary disease, angioplasty, or bypass with hospitalization results in a very strong bond of trust that is formed and must be used to its maximum potential in a therapeutic way by the clinician. With such a captive audience, I began to relish the opportunity to open the door to help patients recognize their personal intellectual-emotional mismatch, to demonstrate that there are feelings and forces operating "under the radar" adversely affecting their physical health. This, in my opinion, is the clinical cardiologist's newest and perhaps most important frontier.

Thus, I had come full circle, from the green medical student salivating at the thought of reading the EKG strip, interpreting it, and instantly making a decision with life or death consequences, to the seasoned clinical cardiologist who can only do so much with his catheters, paddles, defibrillators, and medicines. It *was* the understanding of the human psyche, after all, that was the real key to the puzzle. The cardiology part was relatively easy in comparison. Little did I know that my favorite disease was very often going to be rooted in abnormal human psychology. I had come to learn that it was only in the implementation of the principles of psychology that one could actually cure the patient, not just lower their risk. The answer is inside the patient. The answer is somewhere under the radar.

1. Epidemiology of Coronary Artery Disease: Risk Factors and the Metabolic Syndrome

As you travel through the continuum of coronary disease and its risk factors, human behavior and non-compliance, and operative psychological mechanisms, you must first understand the scope of coronary disease, and the enormity of the problem. We are a manic, over-the-top society—fast-paced, competitive, and expensive. News is at our fingertips, sometimes too extreme to bear witness to. We are over-stimulated. Time is a difficult commodity to accumulate. We are dropping dead from heart attacks and heart disease.

Coronary artery disease (CAD) remains the number one killer of all men and women in the United States annually. In fact, there are more deaths from CAD than from the second, third, fourth, and fifth most common causes of death combined! Annually, CAD results in 600,000 deaths and 1.1 million myocardial infarctions, of which 650,000 are first occurrences. The economic burden of CAD on a yearly basis is 101 billion dollars. While homeland and global security are important priorities of our government and society today, in comparison to our global challenges, you can now see the devastation and expense this disease levies on us, year in and year out. The good news is that there is much we can do about it.

We talk about "risk factors" for the development or progression of coronary artery disease. Risk factors are clinical variables in your personal health profile that put you at higher risk than the general population for contracting the disease. Or, if you already have the disease, not correcting or eliminating ongoing risk factors will likely result in accelerating the progression of your problem. Keep in mind, however, that for those who have not yet contracted the disease, these are only risk factors. They are not actually synonymous with having the disease itself. For example, there are people diagnosed with lung cancer who have never smoked (despite smoking being a potent risk factor for lung cancer), and conversely, there are smokers who never develop lung cancer. Although possessing a risk factor statistically increases your likelihood of getting a particular disease, it is not a guarantee, nor is a perfect risk profile a guarantee that you will remain disease-free. That being said, the message to take home here is that risk factors, especially when they occur in multiples, are potent catalysts in the formation and progression of CAD, and they must be taken very seriously. They have a high statistical correlation with major coronary events and death, and their reduction, even in small increments, has profound effects, improving these unwanted outcomes.

Major risk factors for CAD are:

1. Age
2. Gender (male > female)
3. Family history of premature coronary disease (mother, father, brother or sister having had an MI before age 60)
4. Elevated total cholesterol (> 200 milligrams per deciliter [mg/dL], or > 230 mg/dL, depending on your individual risk profile); or elevated low density lipoprotein cholesterol (LDL) (> 100 mg/dL or > 130 mg/dL, depending on your individual risk profile)
5. Reduced HDL (high density lipoprotein) cholesterol (< 50 mg/dL in females and < 40 mg/dL in males)
6. Tobacco use

Elliot Brown, M.D., F.A.C.C.

7. Hypertension (blood pressure > 140/90 millimeters of mercury [mm Hg])
8. Diabetes mellitus
9. Obesity (Body Mass Index ≥ 25 is overweight, and ≥ 30 is obese)
10. Sedentary lifestyle

It should also be stated that there is a well-known syndrome, the metabolic syndrome, that is a constellation of risk factors pooled together in the same patient. Metabolic syndrome is present if a patient has three of the following five criteria:

1. Abdominal obesity
2. Hypertension
3. Diabetes mellitus
4. Elevated triglyceride level
   (Triglyceride > 150 mg/dL)
5. Low HDL cholesterol level
   (< 50 mg/dL in females and < 40 mg/dL in males)

In addition, there is a theme in cardiovascular prevention that when risk factors occur together in groups such as the ones listed above, they combine to create significantly higher risk than the sum of each of them individually. That's known in medical terms as a "synergistic" effect. Put simply, it's one of those situations where 1 + 1 = 3.

The metabolic syndrome is a unique interplay of hormonal changes that results in a group of patients at very high risk for the complications of atherosclerotic vascular disease, or "hardening of the arteries." So-called "hardening of the arteries" most commonly presents itself in the form of coronary artery disease, cerebrovascular disease (stroke), abdominal aortic aneurysm, or peripheral vascular disease (poor circulation to the limbs, especially lower). The common scenario in our society nowadays is the chronic overeater developing abdominal adipose, or abdominal fat. This increase in weight often increases the person's blood pressure, and now you have 2 out of the 5 criteria: abdominal obesity and hypertension. As a result of changes that take place in the setting of increased abdominal fat, the fat cells produce a certain hormone, cortisol, and also decrease their number of insulin receptors by a process known as "down-regulation." (I'll explain).

When a person ingests certain carbohydrates classified as high glycemic index carbohydrates, blood sugar levels will rise quickly, and insulin is released as a result. Similarly, insulin levels in the bloodstream will also elevate quickly to attempt to lower the blood sugar back to normal. In a typical American diet, which has an overabundance of high glycemic index carbohydrates, the sugar levels rise fast and high, as do the insulin levels. Over time, from repetition of this process, the cells utilizing sugar for energy say to themselves, "Since sugar is so abundant in my surroundings, I don't need so many docking stations (receptors) on my cell membrane for it; I can get all the sugar I need with fewer docking stations." The cell then begins to change by making fewer receptors for insulin to facilitate the passage of glucose from the bloodstream into the cell. This process is called down-regulation of the receptors.

Let's play out what then happens metabolically because of this chemical and functional change induced by a high glycemic index diet: When you eat a carbohydrate meal first thing in the morning after fasting, your blood sugar level rises, and now the insulin that is released in response to the high sugar level has relatively fewer "docking stations" at the site of the cell membrane to allow the sugar to pass into the cell, thereby removing the glucose from the bloodstream. Thus, the sugar hangs around in the blood stream longer, raising blood glucose levels over an inordinately long period of time. This is called glucose intolerance, or adult onset diabetes. A lower number of insulin receptors results in glucose intolerance; put simply, with a decreased number of avenues to pass blood glucose into the cells for use as energy, the patient is less tolerant of a "usual" dietary glucose load. This is the essence of the pathophysiology behind the adult onset diabetic state, or type II diabetes mellitus.

Once frank diabetes is present, lipid abnormalities often ensue in the form of high triglyceride and low HDL cholesterol. This is an encapsulated spectrum of the metabolic syndrome and its pathogenesis. There is a strong interplay among weight, blood pressure, diabetes, and certain lipid disorders. So, in this syndrome, all you have to do is lose weight, which will improve blood pressure, eliminate the abdominal fat pad, and thus reduce the tendency toward diabetes and eliminate the lipid abnormality. Easy as one, two, three, right?

Wrong. The problem arises when the patient first recognizes that there is much he or she can do as an individual to alter the outcome of his or her disease. Modifiable risk factors are risk factors that we can change. Age, for example, is a risk factor we cannot change. On the other hand, weight, the degree or presence of hypercholesterolemia (high cholesterol level), hypertension (high blood pressure), and cigarette smoking can be altered significantly by the patient. By modifying those risk factors that can be altered, the patient will gain statistical advantages that mathematically reduce the risk of poor outcomes in cardiovascular disease. The good news here is that even small steps in the right direction may have profound beneficial effects on any given patient. For example, a 1% decline in LDL cholesterol results in a 1 - 2% decrease in subsequent cardiovascular events. This means if your LDL is lowered from 300 mg/dL to 210 mg/dL, you experience a 30 - 60% decrease in risk of cardiovascular events. A 1% decline in mean blood pressure results in a 2 - 4% decrease in subsequent cardiovascular events. A 1% increase in HDL cholesterol results in 2% and 3% reductions in cardiovascular events in men and women, respectively. In this example, if your HDL level rises from 35 mg/dL to 38.5 mg/dL, you experience a 20 - 30% reduction in risk of cardiovascular events.

Smoking cessation reduces the cardiac event rate by up to 47%. With just one maneuver, there is perhaps nothing more powerful in reducing adverse cardiac events than quitting smoking. Rounding out the prevention strategy involves good glucose control in diabetics, diet and weight control, and an increase in physical activity. Anti-platelet agents (aspirin or clopidogrel), statins, beta-blockers, and ACE-inhibitors (family names of cardiac drugs—ask your doctor if they're appropriate for you) are also pharmacological preventive regimens that statistically improve outcomes in coronary artery disease.

Why is the recognition that I can do so much to alter the outcome of my disease a problem? Because it is here that the human behavior component comes in. It is all up to us. Isn't that what life is really all about anyway? No one is going to do anything for us. My doctor can't stop eating for me. It's a lonely world, in that regard. The realization that we're the only ones who can help ourselves can be quite frightening. It's enough to make one grab a drink, smoke a cigarette, or get lost in a pint of ice cream. It's time to grow up, but I don't want to. Not today. What a fertile ground for the intellectual-emotional gap to thrive. How threatening. No wonder cardiac disease is the number one killer.

2. Rules of the Road

Sometime during my third year in medical school, I had a professor who taught us that as we began to learn about human diseases, we would soon be able to determine if we were "lumpers" or "splitters." Lumpers look at a disease such as coronary artery disease and lump everything together, from the early plaque formation to the blockage to the angina and, finally, to the heart attack. A lumper sees it all as one disease, just different stages, and he will generally recognize and learn the continuum of the disease, memorizing only the small differences at each level. A splitter, in contrast, splits everything up into separate entities and memorizes everything individually. It's a different way of thinking and categorizing things. As you can tell, I am the ultimate lumper, not only starting my continuum with the early plaque, but also going further back to the emotional origin of the disease when the body first develops defense mechanisms to stress. Maladaptive behavior then sets in, gives rise to the metabolic syndrome, and a few decades later, becomes good old-fashioned coronary disease and the ensuing myocardial infarction.

In order to link the emotional states of chronic stress and chronic depression to abnormal bodily physiology, "common denominators" must be recognized. A common denominator, as I call it, is a common chemical or biological pathway in the body that may have multiple origins. Regardless of the origins, these multiple causes converge on the same pathway, resulting in similar processes in the end.

To illustrate this, consider a substance called "tumor necrosis factor" (TNF). TNF is present in both end-stage cancer patients and end-stage congestive heart failure patients. It results in cachexia (pronounced ka-kex-ee-a), that malnourished, muscle-wasting appearance many end-stage patients have. We don't know how to prevent its effect, only that TNF is elevated at these points in the respective diseases. Yet cancer and heart failure are completely different disease processes. If you are a true lumper, you see that there is a unity to it all.

When someone experiences chronic stress, this activates a team of glands called the hypothalamic-pituitary-adrenal axis (HPA axis). These three glands communicate with each other, and under stress they give rise to the secretion, or release, of the hormone cortisol into the bloodstream from the adrenal gland. Thus, people who find that they are suffering from chronic stress, as we will define later in more detail, will have chronically elevated cortisol levels in their bloodstream. Similarly, chronic stress and chronic depression both lead to activation of the sympathetic nervous system which results in elevated levels of the hormone noradrenaline in the blood. The chronic elevation of these hormones, cortisol and noradrenaline, and the overexposure of our organs to them, eventually becomes maladaptive and harmful to the individual. The activation of these hormones may also impart behavioral tendencies that further potentiate the overeating, increase abdominal fat, and fuel the increased cortisol cycle. Thus, there are clearly reactions to chronic stress and depression that occur chemically and behaviorally in our bodies. The maladaptive behavior (smoking, overeating, not exercising, etc.) often occurs as a result of the chronically stressed state. These behaviors serve to reduce stress levels, but only temporarily, which is why they have to be repeated and repeated if they are the only ways one deals with the perceived stress. To complete the continuum, chronic exposure to these behaviors eventually becomes harmful to the individual as the behaviors generally increase cardiovascular risk.

You will see that emotional health has everything to do with how we perceive things, and it is that perception that determines our own individual internal reactions. For those who perceive their environment as depressing or stressful, a physiological change takes place over time that causes chronic exposure to cortisol and noradrenaline. It is also a set-up for chronic behaviors that promote poorer cardiovascular outcomes. The high cortisol and noradrenaline levels eventually contribute to the diabetic state, abdominal obesity, hypertension, and a multiplicity of cardiac risk factors. The emotional factors are also highly associated with behaviors that include non-compliance with medication and medical follow-up, less exercise, and greater consumption of unhealthy foods, cigarettes, and alcohol. This concept of cumulative exposure is well recognized in human medicine. Chances are, after a certain amount of exposure to virtually any stimulus, more harm than good is likely to set in.

So, we now have the link and the pathway through which human psychology meets physical disease. Emotional distress in the form of depression, anxiety, or chronic stress converges in the common denominators: excess cortisol and noradrenaline, which subsequently fuel the atherosclerotic process. If you really want to change outcomes in a physical disease, you must acknowledge the presence of its true origins and delve into them accordingly.

*

I remember sitting in my chair in front of the stage at my medical school graduation. Having a last name that begins with the letter "B" gives you privileges that a Zimmerman can only dream of. I was always in front of the line, or in this case, in the first row at graduation. During one of the many speeches on that sweltering June afternoon, I realized that my internship was now only days away, and as grueling as it appeared academically, it looked ten times tougher physically. This was before the time of the Bell Commission in New York City, which meant that I would have a thirty-six hour shift approximately every four days for the next year.

I thought of the lonely nights in the dingy on-call rooms and of the impending exhaustion. It was at that moment that I remember closing my eyes and praying for the strength to be able to get out of bed when I had to. I thought of all the patients in the hospital and of all their functioning intravenous lines providing a conduit for necessary medication. I realized that if any fell out overnight, I would be paged to go put a new one in, and I sincerely prayed for the strength to be able to handle it physically without getting so tired that I wouldn't care if the line went back in or not. I was afraid that cumulative exposure to sleep deprivation would beat me. Thankfully, it didn't.

So much of our experience involves the concept of cumulative exposure. It's the source of the saying "Everything in moderation." A little bit of something is not bad, but too much can kill you. So goes it with chronically elevated cortisol and noradrenaline levels. Initially, the hormones have a purposeful effect, especially in the acute situation, but over time, when they are chronically elevated, we realize that they become catalysts of many pathologic metabolic processes and of the eventual establishment of overt atherosclerotic vascular disease.

3. Depression and Heart Disease

Depression is a potent risk factor associated with the development of coronary artery disease and MI, and conversely, having a heart attack is a potent risk factor for the development of clinical depression. Thus, the two entities are closely linked, and their close relationship should be recognized well by patients and physicians alike. Besides lowering the quality of one's life, depression increases the risk of a recurrent myocardial infarction and increases mortality rates after a myocardial infarction.

Diagnostic criteria for emotional and psychiatric disorders are defined in the *Diagnostic and Statistical Manual of Mental Disorders, Fourth Edition* (DSM-IV). The diagnostic criteria for major depression are as follows. The patient must report a depressed mood most of the day or loss of interest or pleasure (anhedonia) in most activities, and four or more of the following symptoms for a two-week period:

- significant appetite or weight change
- insomnia or hypersomnia almost daily
- psychomotor agitation or retardation
- fatigue or loss of energy
- inability to concentrate or indecisiveness
- recurrent thoughts of death or suicidal ideation

It is well known that depression may occur along a spectrum, from milder forms such as adjustment reaction with depressive features (quite common after an illness such as an MI) to major depression. The more severe the depression is, obviously, the greater the magnitude and duration of symptoms, and the greater the distress and impairment. Along these lines, there is a graded relationship between depression and coronary artery disease. While milder depression is associated with an increase in adverse events, the more severe the depression becomes, the more potent it becomes as a cardiac risk factor. Above and beyond psychomotor agitation or retardation and loss of energy or fatigue, additional symptoms reported by depressed patients include feelings of worthlessness or guilt. Often depression may be difficult to diagnose given that sleep problems, fatigue, energy loss, and thoughts of death may accompany heart disease as well. The cardiac population often presents the above symptoms, but suicidal thoughts or a sense of worthlessness are not classic hallmarks of heart disease.

In a meta-analysis of various clinical studies, depression has been shown to be a cardiac risk factor as potent as the traditional risk factors, such as smoking, diabetes, and hypertension. In large trials that follow patients with cardiac risk factors along for years, depression is consistently more prevalent in those patients who have suffered an MI than in those who haven't. Major depression develops in approximately 20% of patients after an MI, and is present for some time in up to 33% of such patients. Depression is a concern after an MI not only because it continues to represent a risk factor for the next event, but also because depression is associated with poor compliance with treatment strategies such as completing a cardiac rehabilitation program, making follow-up doctor appointments, or simply compliance with taking necessary medications. Thus, for direct and indirect reasons, depression is a complicating feature for cardiac patients.

*

I was once called to the emergency room to see a forty-six-year-old firefighter with a massive heart attack in progress. He had suffered a cardiac arrest in the ambulance on the way to the hospital, and he was "shocked" back to life with the defibrillator. On my arrival his pain was a "ten out of ten," and his EKG was about as acute as they come. Immediately, arrangements were made to bring him to the cardiac catheterization laboratory, where we performed emergency angioplasty of the infarct-related artery. The heart attack was over, but his long-term problems were just beginning. Unfortunately for our patient, enough time had gone by since the onset of the MI that significant damage had been done to his heart muscle, diminishing its overall pump function quite substantially. The proper medications were prescribed, but following his initial recovery, he could no longer go out on emergency calls and thrive in the profession that he had worked so hard at and loved.

For him, wearing the uniform and going out with his colleagues to fight fires had been his identity and his world. Now, he would most likely be destined to have an inside job, relegated to tasks within the department that were more menial, in his opinion. His personal and professional identity was blown out of the water.

Following the hospitalization, he proceeded to have continual complaints of chest pain and required repeat cardiac catheterization a few months later for symptoms, but the stent we had put in was, in fact, wide open. When it became clear that the heart muscle pump function (ejection fraction—EF) was not going to get any better, it was time to recommend an automatic implantable cardioverter defibrillator (AICD) implant to protect him from another cardiac arrest. This further added to his declining self-image.

Severe depression ensued, and I referred him to a psychiatrist, who immediately began medical therapy and supportive psychotherapy. He went out on extended disability and never bounced back to his previous level of well-being, despite never requiring hospitalization for further chest pain or congestive heart failure (CHF), a common complication of a weak heart muscle. I have not seen him for quite a long time, as he became more and more non-compliant with his follow-up appointments and blood tests to follow his cholesterol level. The confounding issue of depression has influenced this young man so much that he is not getting the healthcare he requires, and he is likely headed for additional trouble down the road.

*

For both the patient and the practitioner, recognition of depression is extremely important. Internists and cardiologists alike must become more comfortable with prescribing SSRIs (selective serotonin reuptake inhibitors) for the treatment of depression. Of the various classifications of antidepressant medications, SSRIs appear to be the safest to use in the presence of heart disease, and they generally do not react adversely with commonly prescribed cardiac medications. For milder forms of depression, reassurance and supportive psychotherapy are often all that is necessary.

The majority of cardiac patients experiencing anxiety and depression early after a cardiac event improve steadily within the first six months to one year, unlike our firefighter patient. When symptoms of depression are severe or become chronic, a referral to a psychiatrist is often in order. If the primary clinician (the cardiologist, or sometimes the internist) reserves psychiatric referral for this small population of patients, he or she will enjoy a great deal of success in treating many degrees of depression after a significant cardiac event. In addition, the patient who has been managed in this fashion is more likely to agree to seek psychiatric help after initial efforts have not been entirely successful.

I have found that discussing referral to a mental health professional with a patient immediately after a cardiac event is often met with skeptical eyes and refusal. In the majority of cases to which I have attended, however, patients are willing to confront their emotional issues with the cardiologist and to determine for themselves what improvements can be made with simple recognition, supportive conversation, and in some cases, the above combined with an SSRI medication. When these strategies are exhausted, symptoms are usually significant enough for the patient to seek relief with a mental health professional. Clinical situations that have become most closely associated with the development of depression include myocardial infarction, bypass surgery, angioplasty, cardiac catheterization, and implantation of an AICD.

The cardiologist, having taken the patient through any or all of the above scenarios, is likely to be the one person in the world whom the patient will trust with virtually any aspect of his physical or mental health. It is therefore crucial that the cardiologist be comfortable with the recognition and management of depression in this setting, and for the patient to become comfortable with the recognition and confession of these symptoms and feelings as well. This is a unique opportunity the cardiologist has to really help the patient heal after the trauma he or she has suffered. Cardiologists historically have been quite comfortable with recognizing and addressing maladaptive behaviors in the realms of overeating, sedentary lifestyles, and cigarette smoking. However, diagnosis and treatment of psychosocial risk factors such as depression, anxiety, mental stress, and the like have not classically fallen into the realm of clinical cardiology training. Thus, most cardiologists have limited experience and familiarity with these psychological deficits. This has given rise to the general feeling that it is not within the purview of cardiologists to address these issues given that they are not trained mental health professionals. I suggest that these entities *are* within the cardiologist's scope. Just as the internist, who can recognize hypertension, should begin a treatment plan and reserve the most challenging patients for sub-specialist referral, we cardiologists should become more familiar with psychosocial risk factors because of their intimate relationship with coronary artery disease.

Simply adding a few open-ended questions about sleeping and eating habits to the history during a patient visit is helpful. Similarly, questions concerning feelings of hopelessness or lack of interest in activities that have previously brought the patient pleasure help give insight about levels of depression in a given individual.

A confounding issue is time. The reality of today's health care climate, from the physician's perspective, is an industry of ever-declining reimbursement from insurance companies, ever-increasing overhead from employee wages and the cost of supplies, rising malpractice premiums, and rising health insurance premiums for their personnel. Therefore, the time spent with each individual patient becomes a major factor with respect to the physician's ability to produce enough to ensure that his or her practice can maintain itself fiscally.

Regardless, there are ways to work within the system and incorporate some effective strategies into the practice in order to maximize the physician's therapeutic ability. While patients in a busy cardiology office are often scheduled every fifteen minutes, some patients only require very quick visits that essentially consist of an inquiry about a medicine change or a follow-up examination to check if the lungs are clear. Some time can be generated by seeing such follow-up appointments expeditiously, thus leaving additional time for more complex patients. In addition, if a patient who has difficult psychosocial issues is identified, more frequent visits are often a good solution to the time problem. This works well for two reasons: It gives the patient and physician more time to talk in depth, and it also ensures that during the patient's most difficult and vulnerable clinical period, he or she is being seen more often, which can be very therapeutic for the patient. Remember, most cardiac patients who experience depression after a cardiac event will have significant improvement over the ensuing six months, so this strategy of more frequent office visits for any individual patient is short-lived in the grand scheme of things.

In short, depression is a potent risk factor for poor cardiac outcomes and may precede or follow the initial cardiac event. Physicians and patients alike must recognize this and look out for depression wherever it may be hiding. The cardiologist is often the one health care professional who is most likely to be in a position to recognize when depression is present, and he or she has a golden opportunity to do a great service to his or her patient by becoming familiar with the recognition and treatment of its mild, moderate, or more severe forms. Once embarking on a treatment plan, referral to a mental health professional may be reserved for only the most challenging cases.

4. Psychosocial Stress and Heart Disease

There are two general categories of psychosocial factors that surface as promoters of adverse cardiac events. The first is the group called "affective disorders," which includes depression, anxiety disorders, hostility, and anger. The scope of this section is to discuss the second category, "chronic stressors." In the cardiac literature, this category is specifically made up of low social support, low socioeconomic status, work stress, marital stress, and caregiver strain. One might look at this list and think that everyone has at least one of these stressors in their lives, so is everyone doomed to have one or more of these entities on their cardiac risk list and be headed for an MI? No. While most of the population has some type of stress in their life, it is important to realize that it is not the presence of the stress per se that is so detrimental; it is what the patient does with that stress internally that fuels (or doesn't fuel) the atherosclerosis fire.

Yes, our lives in this frenetic world are full of all kinds of stress. But how people perceive their own stress makes all the difference in how it gets played out clinically with regard to their mental and physical health. Earlier, we touched on how the hormones noradrenaline and cortisol can become the catalysts of the atherosclerotic disease process when chronically elevated as a result of metabolic changes that take place in the body. As we will see later in more detail, maladaptation to these substances is the common denominator that results from affective disorders and chronic stressors gone unchecked. It is the perception of the individual that determines how the external stressor will be interpreted, and thus how it translates physiologically in any given patient.

A great example of this falls into the category of caregiver strain. With our population aging, the incidence of dementia is on the rise, and Alzheimer's dementia comprises 60 - 80% of this group. Baby boomers are getting older, and these figures will only increase with time. While dementia is devastating to the patient, it likely takes the same or an even greater toll on the caregiver, who is usually the spouse or a child. Initially, cognitive dysfunction (dementia) may declare itself in social situations by inappropriate behavior or conversation. Another common warning sign is frustration in the home with regard to the inability to complete common tasks like balancing a checkbook, or requiring repetition of verbal cues in order to stay focused on routine chores and scheduled plans for the day. It is essentially a defect in short-term memory at this point. As the process progresses, independence is impaired and eventually lost by the patient; from the spouse's point of view it feels like having a child to take care of all over again. The only problem is that it is easier to care for a child when you are twenty-five years old than when you're seventy-five years old.

In one study, caregiving for an ill or disabled spouse over a four-year period demonstrated a twofold increased risk for having an adverse cardiac event. But that is not the entire picture. In this study, there was no information about the perceived strain experienced by the care giver. Research suggests that meaningful and altruistic experiences can be a health benefit, and thus if one attaches such sentiment to their caregiving, he or she may not be at as high a risk as the study initially indicated. When caregivers are divided into groups based on whether or not they experience emotional strain during care giving, only those reporting strain associated with their role had an increased death rate when followed up.

Therefore, it is possible that those caregivers who perceive a meaningful or altruistic feeling toward their role with the ill or disabled spouse don't internalize strain as do those who feel encumbered by their newfound burden. In the former situation, the internal metabolic changes that would result in the increased noradrenaline and cortisol levels never takes place, and good health is maintained without the adverse cardiac outcomes. This is why it is important to understand that it is not the removal of all stress that is the goal, but learning about how we internalize or perceive the stress that makes all the difference in our health outcomes. The good news is that if we find ourselves reacting to our external stressors in unhealthy ways, we have an opportunity to work on our reactivity and alter our perceptions in order to ensure better long term outcomes. It is through this nurturing of our mental health that we can truly achieve optimal physical health.

Human beings are social animals, and social support is an important ingredient in living a healthy life. High levels of social support are associated with physical and emotional well-being, and low levels are just the opposite—associated with poorer health outcomes. Suicide rates are higher among those individuals who are described as "loners," and cultures that integrate members into social circles have been shown to suffer a lower occurrence of suicide than those that do not. Social support consists of many factors, including the size, structure, and frequency of contact an individual has with a given social network such as a religious or civic group one may belong to. In addition, the amount of resources any individual receives (and the perception of how satisfying that is for the individual) from such a group is also an important factor. This includes help accomplishing personal tasks, economic support, advice that can be received from peers, or emotional support, including feelings of belonging and being loved. An inadequacy in any or all of these areas is associated with increased cardiac mortality. Other factors that contribute to poorer cardiac outcomes in this arena include living alone, lacking a confidant, or suffering from social isolation.

Under the envelope of socioeconomic status are characteristics such as occupation, financial status, and social status. There exists an inverse relationship between socioeconomic status and adverse cardiac outcomes. In other words, those at higher levels of socioeconomic status have lower risk and those at a lower socioeconomic status have higher risk. Low socioeconomic status is unfortunately associated with poorer health habits and a higher frequency of classic cardiac risk factors. In addition, this group experiences more financial difficulties, poorer housing, less opportunity for education, and greater difficulty in the health care system. They also are likely to have less job security and job latitude and often are required to perform more physically demanding and repetitive work. All of these factors lend themselves to poorer cardiac outcomes.

It has been shown that metabolic dysfunction in the form of increased cortisol levels accompanies chronic stress, and increased dysfunction of this hormonal system is observed as socioeconomic status of an individual declines. It is this physiologic observation that essentially suggests that low socioeconomic status in and of itself may be considered a chronic psychological stressor.

There are two major areas in the workplace that seem to be associated with worsening clinical outcomes. In the job strain model described by Karasek *et al.,* individuals who experience high job demand but low job latitude suffer significant emotional stress. This is the situation in which there exists excessive routine work with a pervasiveness of rigid confinement and no outlet for creativity. Effort-reward imbalance, another form of chronic job stress that has been described, suggests that excessive demand on the job (either imposed by the employer or self-imposed by one's internal drive to be productive) predicts adverse events when it is out of proportion to financial remuneration, self-esteem, opportunity to advance vertically, or ability to obtain job security.

*

I recently consulted a 44-year-old female who was complaining of a few months' history of chest pain not specifically related to exertion or relieved by rest. This is called atypical chest pain because it may represent coronary artery disease but is not a typical presentation of it. She was an accomplished athlete, appeared quite fit, and was upset that such a "healthy" person with good habits could be having chest pain and find herself in a cardiologist's office.

She had a very high-level job in law enforcement, and recently had endured a significant change in the personnel to whom she was immediately responsible. After six years at a position she loved and was quite successful at, she found herself limited by the constraints of her newfound administration. Initially, we focused on the change in her perception about how she now fits in at the workplace. It was clear that she was experiencing significant effort-reward imbalance, and it was not agreeing with her at all.

Given that she had a few cardiac risk factors, including a family history of premature coronary disease, I did order a stress test to rule out this as the cause; the majority of the time, however, was spent delving into her psychosocial stress. She realized that she needed to work on her reactivity at the workplace and she began psychotherapy as well in order to learn as much as she could about herself. Thus, she initiated the process of taking things into her own hands to effect therapeutic change. This is a great example of how we can be proactive for ourselves and adjust how we perceive our surroundings. It is not wise to wait for our environment to change every time we come across hard psychological times. This "healthy" side to this patient will undoubtedly serve her well and will clearly lower her statistical risk of a poor cardiac outcome. She is one patient who immediately understood that for her, the answer was somewhere under the radar.

*

Finally, marital stress is another chronic stressor that can have significant physiologic effects. One report indicates that, following myocardial infarction, women who returned home to significant perceived marital stress demonstrated a higher frequency of recurrent cardiac events during the ensuing five years than did their counterparts who did not suffer the same marital stress. Another study identified a greater amount of subclinical atherosclerosis and greater acceleration of it over time among "healthy" women who reported marital dissatisfaction. Thus, similar to other forms of chronic stress, marital stress in particular may be viewed as an atherogenic process.

It is important to keep in mind that although I have discussed depression and chronic stressors as independent variables (this goes along with the "splitter" mentality I discussed earlier), in reality, most of the time these entities are clustered (lumped) together in any given individual. It is hard to come from a low socioeconomic status, have no job latitude, suffer from financial pressure and marital difficulties, and not have some depression as well. The take-home message is that virtually any life situation that results in chronic stress or depression represents significant psychosocial risk. The common denominator as we will see in great detail in the next chapter is that these psychosocial risk factors, when present chronically, will invariably result in maladaptation of our internal "stress response" and thus fuel the atherogenic process. In addition, the presence of these psychosocial risk factors are also associated with a greater incidence of unhealthy lifestyles and behaviors which often add to the patient's list of traditional cardiac risk factors, thereby further contributing to worsened cardiac outcomes.

Thus, it is critical to understand that "I have too much stress" is no longer an excuse for brazen noncompliance. There is much opportunity to work on the way you react to your environment, and you now have the insight as to why that is the case. When you react to your environment and perceive it as chronically stressful or when you have untreated depression or anxiety, the nervous system is affected in such a way as to chronically increase noradrenaline and cortisol levels. These biochemicals have damaging effects on your metabolism and, eventually, on your vascular system. It is therefore how you deal with your perceived stress that will make all the difference as to whether this chemical change is going to take place and subsequently do you harm.

The goal is to possess a certain emotional resilience that will foster your ability to avoid those emotionally harmful perceptions that invariably result in your going down this deleterious physiological road—a road that will eventually come to a dead end in the form of adverse cardiac events. The desired emotional resilience can be obtained through initially recognizing that you are not handling your emotional stress in a healthy manner, and then gaining the courage to talk about it and work on it in a therapeutic setting. It is this recognition that is the key first step toward health and success. While the cardiologist is not a trained psychologist, it should be well within the repertoire of the clinician to assist in the unveiling of the patient's intellectual-emotional mismatch, and in many cases to initiate therapeutic discussions.

Once patients recognize within themselves the ability to see "under the radar," then and only then will they begin to "own" their problems. By taking ownership of their emotional difficulties, they often become quite eager to begin to do something about them because they then know too much and can't go back and continue to hide in their previous dysfunctional "comfort zones." It's important to remember that while this may be a seemingly painful and difficult undertaking, it is all part of human nature, and you can only be commended for trying to improve your coping skills and become emotionally and physically healthier.

5. The Knee Bone is Connected to the Shin Bone

To this point, I have alluded to "common physiologic denominators" that represent the metabolic process by which maladaptive changes take place within our bodies and cause overt disease. The purpose of this section is to describe in greater detail the specific ways in which this occurs, so that you will see how psychosocial risk factors have such significant physical ramifications. The saying "Died of a broken heart" may be generations old, but it is not until recently that the physiology behind this notion has become well understood. The two major players in this arena are the hormones noradrenaline (of which adrenaline is a by-product) and cortisol. A hormone is a chemical secreted into the bloodstream that performs an action in some area of the body other than that from which it came.

For the purpose of this discussion, we will divide the nervous system into two components, the voluntary and the involuntary. For example, voluntary actions include picking up this book or eating, but the central nervous system's involuntary part, called the autonomic nervous system, deals with functions that we don't actively think about, such as heart rate, respiratory rate, and the like. The autonomic nervous system is a complex balance between the sympathetic nervous system and the parasympathetic nervous system. The sympathetic nervous system controls our "fight or flight" response. In other words, when fully activated, it prepares us to fight a physical threat or run away in order to survive. While we don't often have to confront a predator in the wild, a common illustration of this component of our nervous system is the scenario in which a woman picks up a car in order to remove her trapped child. The parasympathetic nervous system opposes that function, and when dominating the balance, promotes rest, sleep, digestion, and more vegetative processes. The main messenger, or hormone, of the sympathetic nervous system is noradrenaline, and its counterpart in the parasympathetic nervous system is acetylcholine. We will mainly be concerned with the sympathetic nervous system here.

Cortisol comes from the adrenal glands, which are small glands that reside on the north poles of each of our kidneys. They are controlled directly by the pituitary gland, which takes its orders from and is connected to a structure in the brain called the hypothalamus (HPA-axis). The sympathetic nervous system is chronically overactivated in states of depression, chronic stress, and anxiety.

Sympathetic nervous system activation by virtue of the effects of noradrenaline and adrenaline, among other things, results in increased heart rate, blood pressure, and oxygen demand from heart muscle cells. When heart muscle cells demand oxygen and the supply is diminished, as in coronary artery disease, a mismatch occurs and results in a condition called myocardial ischemia, which can become detrimental to the heart's functioning. The sympathetic nervous system also activates the HPA-axis, resulting in chronically elevated cortisol levels. Under normal circumstances, when an individual is exposed to acute stress, that individual is wired to respond appropriately in order to survive. Noradrenaline results in greater skeletal muscle blood flow so the individual may perform whatever physical activity is necessary to get away from a stressor such as a predator. In addition, heart rate increases to provide more cardiac output, and the HPA-axis is stimulated. The hypothalamus and pituitary glands then send a messenger to the adrenal glands, asking them to pump out more cortisol. The increased blood cortisol in the acute setting, among other things, results in maintaining blood glucose levels in order to provide energy for the stress response. Increased appetite is also a result of increased cortisol levels. Once the acute stressor is no longer a perceived threat, and blood glucose levels have risen, it is the elevated concentration of sugar in the blood stream that signals the hypothalamus and pituitary glands to shut off their instructions to the adrenal glands. The "feedback loop" is shut off, or completed, and the acute stress response is over.

What happens in chronic stress? Clearly, the sympathetic nervous system is chronically activated, and this results in constant signaling to the adrenal glands to keep pumping out cortisol into the bloodstream. Since cortisol stimulates appetite, and its goal is to keep enough glucose around in the bloodstream to fuel the extra energy needed for the stress response, carbohydrate craving by the individual results. What follows is a chronic desire to ingest carbohydrates, which in turn increases blood sugar levels, and eventually results in abdominal obesity by virtue of the increased caloric intake that accompanies this process. Note that unlike the acute stress response, which is the evolutionary function of the HPA-axis, the signaling by the brain to the adrenal gland is never shut off in the chronic stress response because the individual continues to perceive stress on a chronic basis.

In the case of chronic stress, elevated blood sugar levels result from ingesting high glycemic index carbohydrates that try to eventually diminish the signal from the pituitary to the adrenal glands, and subsequently shut off the cycle. However, since the chronic stress never goes away completely and is therefore always present to some extent, the process is allowed to continue. Stress is perceived, cortisol levels rise, and the carbohydrate craving again is the result. Over time, caloric intake becomes overly abundant and the patient develops abdominal obesity, which results in hypertension, and insulin resistance, better known as diabetes mellitus. There you have the physiological basis of the psychological contribution to the very high risk metabolic syndrome.

Patients who have significant psychosocial risk factors realize intellectually that they are promoting an unhealthy lifestyle once they are in this situation. They try to diet properly when "read the riot act" by their physician, but often succumb to their carbohydrate cravings. This can set up a cycle of repeated failure, alterations in self-image, loss of confidence, and even loss of self-esteem. If you understand this process, you will realize that it may not be the patient's fault entirely. There is truly a physio-logic cause to the carbohydrate craving. It is not that the patients are simply weak individuals. Their bodies are actually "telling" them to continue to eat carbohydrates. A vicious cycle is set up that spins out of their control.

The key is to understand that the psychosocial factors of de-pression, chronic stress, anxiety, etc., are at work here under the radar. Identifying these and working on how the particular pa-tient deals with the given stress is the most effective and long-term way to put an end to the never-ending feedback loop in the body that the chronic stressor causes. This is perhaps the only way once and for all to shut off the chronic stress response that results in sympathetic overactivation and continued overstimula-tion of the HPA-axis. Education about shifting the carbohydrate choices to a low glycemic index diet rather than the more common high glycemic index diet is often a good start and a short term solution while the patient begins working on dimin-ishing the magnitude of the psychosocial stress.

There is no one system in our body that works independent of the others, and this includes the system of the emotions. For the longest time, traditional medical doctors and mental health professionals have behaved as though the two fields are separate species, one discipline that deals with the tangible, observable physical maladies and another that deals with emotions and the more abstract. Often the gap that exists between these specialties is so wide that there is rarely a conversation between the two, even when patients are shared in common. It is high time that cardiologists and patients see the global view that combines emo-tion and organic disease, and understand how the two entities are so intimately linked. The relationship between the cardiologist and the cardiac patient is the ideal scenario for this interplay to take place, and when it does, the patient is all the better for it. The human heart and human emotion are deeply rooted together, and the recognition of this relationship is the first step toward truly embarking on a long term cure for the patient.

6. Life after Heart Disease

To this point, we have emphasized how psychosocial risk factors translate into potent cardiovascular risk factors for the formation of atherosclerosis and overt coronary artery disease. Identification and management of these problems before coronary disease becomes clinically apparent is crucial, for the many reasons stated above. Unfortunately, not all patients come to clinical attention before their first MI, and not all patients can prevent an MI despite careful risk factor management. Unlike chronic diseases such as emphysema, AIDS, and many cancers, coronary artery disease is characterized by sudden unexpected events that are quite frightening, dramatic, and profound to the patient. In between episodes, the patient usually feels entirely well.

Anxiety and depression are very common after a myocardial infarction. As already indicated, for most patients the emotional distress associated with such an event is relatively short lived. However, for a significant portion, symptoms of anxiety and/or depression may last for many months or years after the index event. Often anxiety and depression will exist together, although there seems to be a tendency for anxiety levels to be highest early on after a heart attack, with depression coming later.

An entity not commonly discussed in the post-MI literature is post traumatic stress disorder (PTSD). There is emerging data that this anxiety disorder is more prevalent than once thought in the post-MI population. Initially studied in the context of enduring war or a natural disaster, PTSD is also present when an individual suffers a serious injury or threat of death and as a result experiences intense fear, horror, or helplessness. PTSD may present itself in one of three ways among patients: re-experiencing symptoms (includes thoughts or flashbacks, or preoccupation with the event); avoidance and numbing symptoms (avoiding any cues that remind the individual of the event); or physiological hyperarousal. Acute MI is a medical entity that psychologically may mimic an environmental traumatic event, and thus is a likely culprit to cause PTSD in the cardiac patient. Cardiac arrest, defibrillation, and cardiac catheterization are other cardiac events that have been shown to represent psychologically similar distress to the patient and are associated with PTSD.

The DSM-IV definition of post traumatic stress disorder is as follows: The patient experienced, witnessed, or was confronted with an event that involved the threat of death or serious injury or a threat to the physical integrity of the self. The patient's response involved intense fear, helplessness, or horror.

The traumatic event is re-experienced in one or more ways:

- recurrent and distressing recollections of the event
- recurrent dreams of the event
- feeling as if the traumatic event were recurring
- distress when exposed to cues that resemble the event
- physiological reactivity when exposed to cues that resemble the event

Persistent avoidance of stimuli associated with the trauma and numbing of general responsiveness must include three or more of the following:

- avoidance of thoughts, feelings, or conversations associated with the trauma
- avoidance of activities, places, or people that are reminders of the trauma
- feeling detached or estranged from others
- restricted range of mood
- sense of foreshortened future

Persistent symptoms of arousal must include two or more of the following:

- difficulty falling or staying asleep
- irritability or angry outbursts
- difficulty concentrating
- hyper-vigilance
- excessive startled responses

PTSD may be present in 8% of patients three to six months following MI, and depending on the study, may range from 8% to 25% of patients six to eighteen months following MI or CABG surgery. PTSD has also been reported in patients who have received automatic implantable cardioverter-defibrillators (AICDs). This disorder comes with functional impairment in some, and is often accompanied by high levels of anxiety, depression, and hostility. The dysfunction observed in some patients may go so far as the impairment of social functioning, difficulty or inability in returning to work, and diminished quality of life.

Since avoidance of stimuli associated with the trauma of the index occurrence is a characteristic of PTSD, patients' compliance with treatment may be greatly affected, as taking medication and going to doctor appointments serve to remind the patient of the stressful event. This behavior would obviously worsen expected cardiac outcomes in a post-MI population. While hyperarousal in patients experiencing war or natural disaster trauma results in patients perhaps scanning their environment hyper-vigilantly, heart disease is internal, and these patients become hypersensitive to physical clues they may experience. Post-MI PTSD patients are more likely to overreact to a perceived change in their breathing, heart rate, or various chest sensations, and to respond to internal sensations in a hyper-vigilant manner. For this reason, they often become recurrent users of emergency medical services such as ambulances and emergency rooms.

PTSD patients have heightened sympathetic nervous system arousal, which, as you are now well aware, sets the chronic stress reaction off, resulting in the damaging effects of noradrenaline and cortisol already discussed. In addition, because patients become so frightened by the initial event, worsened cardiac outcomes are also a result of lower tolerance of physical exercise for fear it will trigger another cardiac event. Studies indicate that anxious individuals have higher rates of hypertension, hypercholesterolemia, and diabetes. They are also known to have higher rates of cigarette smoking and alcohol abuse.

Another entity well described in the coronary artery disease population is panic disorder, the definition of which is as follows: The patient must report recurrent panic attacks, followed by one month of persistent concern about additional panic attacks, worry about the implications or consequences of a panic attack, or significant change in behavioral routine related to the attacks. A panic attack is a discrete period of intense fear or discomfort in which at least four of the following symptoms develop abruptly and reach a peak with ten minutes:

- palpitations
- sweating
- trembling or shaking
- shortness of breath
- choking
- chest pain
- nausea or abdominal distress
- dizziness or faintness
- derealization (feeling of unreality) or depersonalization (being detached from oneself)
- fear of losing control or going crazy
- fear of dying
- paresthesia
- chills or hot flushes

Palpitations, sweating, shortness of breath, choking, chest pain, nausea, and dizziness or faintness are all features shared in common with true cardiac presentations. Cardiologists are often called to see patients for any of the above, but rarely make the diagnosis of panic disorder. The challenge is that many patients with coronary disease may have panic disorder or an anxiety disorder in addition, making the differentiation between one malady and another quite challenging. Just as with other psychosocial risk factors and emotional disorders, there is considerable overlap, and patients with panic disorder may also demonstrate features of PTSD and/or depression.

*

To illustrate this point brings to mind a fifty-seven-year-old female I recently evaluated as a second opinion consultant. She had a history of anxiety disorder and metabolic syndrome. She had recently presented to the hospital unexpectedly with an acute MI and had a stent placed in the culprit artery almost immediately, suffering a small to medium amount of permanent damage. The cardiologist discharged her home after two or three days, stating that the other arteries were clear, and reassured her that she would do just fine. In addition to having been shaken from the event emotionally, upon returning home she began to complain that at night she couldn't breathe well, especially when lying down, and that sometimes she had to sit up to make her breathing easier.

Upon follow-up with her cardiologist, she was reassured that cardiologically she was just fine, and was given Xanax, an anti-anxiety medication, for her post-MI anxiety. Despite this, her nights became a time of apprehension and fear, and her subjective symptoms of shortness of breath just wouldn't improve. Her anxiety levels continued to rise, and all the while her subjective symptoms didn't go away.

After approximately two weeks of this nighttime pattern, she saw me for a second opinion. Echocardiography at that time showed that her mitral valve (one of four valves in the heart) was severely leaking, which is a known complication of the type of heart attack she had. She was having daily recurrent bouts of congestive heart failure due to her leaking valve. It became obvious to me that she needed mitral valve surgery for repair or replacement of the valve. Because of this patient's history of anxiety, there was a significant delay in her proper medical diagnosis, which could have resulted in her demise. Following corrective surgery, she has done well, and is on her way toward feeling like herself again and moving on with her life. This is a perfect example of a patient being stereotyped by her emotional history in which due medical diligence was not used. It illustrates a complicated case demonstrating that emotional issues may travel together with bona fide medical problems. While it is important to address the emotional issues, it is never a substitute for first ruling out organic medical problems in every patient.

✶

As an aid to the cardiologist in screening patients for anxiety, PTSD, and depression, there exist questionnaires that patients can fill out, which can alert both the physician and the patient that any combination of these disorders may be a confounding factor. The State-Trait Anxiety Inventory (STAI), the Posttraumatic Diagnostic Scale (PDS), and the Beck Depression Inventory (BDI) are well known and widely used for this purpose. These tools are not commonly used by cardiologists, but may become useful clinically as cardiologists become more involved in screening their patients for the presence of anxiety, PTSD, and depression. Given some of the time constraints in today's private practice setting, described above, these questionnaires may be given to patients by allied health personnel prior to their visit with the cardiologist, thus helping identify those individuals who may benefit from the initiation of treatment, or when appropriate, referral to mental health professionals. Familiarity with these tools at a minimum can give the clinician a sample of the key ingredients to each disorder and can provoke thought about open-ended questions that can become part of regular history-taking.

Awareness of the effect of emotional unrest on patients doesn't stop with evaluating patients' risk factors before coronary disease presents itself. Once coronary artery disease occurs, there remain many affective disorders in addition to chronic stressors that may continue to fuel the atherosclerotic process, guaranteeing poor outcomes for patients. Depression, post traumatic stress disorder, generalized anxiety disorder, and panic disorder are four such entities that should be actively screened for and treated when present in coronary disease populations. These are common maladies seen in the population of patients with heart disease, and they markedly affect cardiac outcomes for the worse. While we know these entities are adverse to the well-being of our patients, current research is under way to conclusively determine if treatment of these disorders per se improves outcomes statistically. While it would make sense intuitively, more data is necessary so that we may continue to practice evidence-based medicine and not make clinical decisions based solely on our intuitions.

7. Is There Any Good News?

Friedrich Nietzsche said, "That which does not kill us can only make us stronger." Are there psychological features of individuals that may counterbalance negative emotions and impart emotional health and well-being on individuals? Resilience has been looked at in those demonstrating the capacity to bounce back from a trauma and to withstand hardship. Characteristics of individuals with resilience include active problem solving ability, a sense of control, optimism, ability to adapt to change, ability to handle unpleasant emotions, self-confidence, initiative, humor, insight, and creativity. While it is hard to measure any of these features of one's personality, perhaps their suggestion could provoke psychological goals for those less able to bounce back. Concentrating on those virtues that promote good health is a way to enhance one's psychological strength and outlook.

Vitality has been described as a key component toward possessing resilience, as well. It is characterized by a presence of energy and enthusiasm and a sense of "aliveness." In addition, the emotions of joy and interest are fueled by a sense of purpose and self-worth. These emotions have been described to have a feedback on each other such that vitality enhances the emotions of joy and interest, and joy and interest along with purpose and self-worth fuel the feeling of vitality. Both combine to give the individual a sense of resilience, or emotional competence—the ability to handle adversity and sustain emotional flexibility following difficult times.

While the biological basis upon which these positive emotions may operate has not been fully worked out, there exists data in the literature indicating that positive emotions can enhance immune function. Along these lines exists a large study of men whose cardiac outcomes were looked at as they were stratified into groups categorized as optimistic, pessimistic and neutral by responses to a questionnaire. The results suggest a relationship between levels of optimism and better cardiac outcomes, with the optimistic group demonstrating only half the cardiac risk of the pessimistic group. Finally, data also exists showing a strong relationship between positive emotions and longevity in a large group of nuns followed long term. While this is not a complete proof of how important possessing positive emotions are toward achieving good health, these are certainly strong suggestions that must be taken seriously and represent a fertile area for future research.

To illustrate this concept on a more practical level, after a myocardial infarction, there are perhaps two major paths a given patient can take psychologically. We have demonstrated well the scenario in which emotional factors are overwhelming and increase the potential for unhealthy behaviors and lifestyle, which will inevitably promote further illness. The converse of this is the patient who truly receives the "wake-up call" and is able to make major lifestyle changes that enhance health and have a major effect on how coronary artery disease will ultimately express itself. Many patients adopt exercise, make dietary changes, give up smoking, and claim they have become healthier than they have ever been. This level of success then feeds back upon itself, instilling a sense of well-being, self-purpose, and self-esteem. While it seems easy to pick intellectually which scenario you would want to fall into, beware that there may be many emotional obstacles in your way. Intellect is not the problem. Your emotions may just not be there…yet. If you find this is the case, then you have some degree of intellectual-emotional mismatch and are a prime candidate to begin looking at what is lurking under the radar.

*

Shortly after I completed my cardiology training in 1994 and went into my present cardiology practice, I attended to a sixty-two-year-old retired pilot admitted to the hospital for respiratory failure and requiring a respirator for water in his lungs (pulmonary edema). He had a history of hypertension that was not well controlled, and he required a few days of intravenous medications and diuretics in order to relieve him of the fluid overloaded state and wean him off the respirator. An echocardiogram done at the bedside demonstrated that his heart was very weak, which was a new finding for him. Cardiac catheterization proved to be negative for coronary artery disease, indicating that his arteries were wide open, and the heart muscle dysfunction was attributed to severe hypertensive heart disease; he was to be treated medically. Based on his clinical criteria at that time, he had about a 50% chance of surviving five years.

As a cardiology fellow, I participated in a clinical trial prior to the FDA approval of a new heart failure drug, Carvedilol. This beta-blocker medication markedly improves survival in CHF, and over time can actually improve ejection fraction. Once this patient became medically stable, I obtained permission from the drug company for compassionate use of Carvedilol, given that it was not yet fully approved by the FDA. Luckily for him, he was one of the first patients of many to come who would markedly benefit from the long-term use of this highly effective heart failure agent.

The rest was up to him. He abandoned eating food containing sodium, took his medication as prescribed, followed his weight carefully, and made every follow-up appointment he ever scheduled. He eagerly looked forward to follow-up echocardiograms to see if his heart was getting stronger, and he never had high blood pressure again by virtue of his newfound compliance. Despite lower back problems, he maintained as active a lifestyle as he could, and he has exceeded medical expectations with his steady improvement. While his EF has never returned to normal, it has improved significantly, and he is alive today enjoying his four grandchildren, all of whom were born after his initial hospitalization. He is a perfect example of what patient participation can do to improve one's outcome and enjoyment of a satisfying, long life.

8. Bridging the Intellectual-Emotional Gap

What can we do together as physicians and patients to identify emotional factors and improve on them so they won't be as harmful as when they are permitted to continue unchecked?

First and foremost, it is important to keep in mind that small changes may have large outcomes, and goal setting must be appropriate for each individual patient. Those patients with poor social support systems will benefit from being referred to programs or activities that provide greater social support and structure. Exercise programs and activities must be tailored to a given individual's capability, and when starting off, it is important to begin by taking small steps that will give positive reinforcement. It took many years to develop the coronary artery disease, and it will not go away in one month at the gym. Sometimes just getting on the treadmill and walking without an incline for five minutes 3 times per week is the right start. It gets a new routine going, and just starting this practice is likely to be a positive experience for many reasons, both psychologically and physically. The old axiom "No pain, no gain" does not apply to cardiac patients and maintaining good mental and physical health.

Frequent office follow-ups in the beginning may enhance patient compliance and foster structure and support for any given patient. Often it may be useful to have patients assist in creating their own individualized plans rather than dictating tasks and goals to them. Most office practices have a wealth of information available to patients to help them learn about their condition. Many physicians refer patients to nutritional counseling, and this may be another way of developing supervised dietary instruction with appropriate goal setting and progress tracking. It is also another supportive relationship the patient can form along the path to recovery. Relaxation training in the form of audiotapes, therapeutic massage, imagery, and deep breathing may be practiced regularly, and stress management is imperative in the form of involvement in hobbies, yoga, music, pets, or other pleasurable activities.

In addition, I attempt to enroll all of my post-MI and post-open-heart patients in a cardiac rehabilitation program. Cardiac rehabilitation offers the patient many of the above opportunities to help them get well. I am most impressed with the physical therapists and nurses I have met who dedicate their careers to helping my patients with their cardiac rehabilitation. They are well schooled in many of the psychosocial factors discussed above, as well as in exercise physiology and nutrition. The programs offer excellent structure and good medical follow-up for the patients. Individuals learn how to exercise on modern equipment and what their bodies are capable of while under the watch of a cardiac monitor. These programs are also a place where patients can develop relationships with each other, which serves as a great support system and sounding board in which they can discuss personal experiences and concerns.

Along the lines of evidence-based medicine, cardiac rehabilitation programs have been shown to improve mortality rates in those patients who attend and complete a three-month program. When exercise and risk factor education are combined, there is a statistically significant reduction in myocardial infarction rates. For this reason, most if not all health insurance companies provide full coverage for cardiac rehabilitation in post-MI and post-open-heart patients.

Most of the above suggestions may be accomplished in or around today's cardiology practices. For patients manifesting frank anxiety, panic, PTSD, or depression, talking is an extremely effective tool for recognition and initial reassurance. Medical therapy, when necessary, may be accomplished with SSRIs, and for more severe or chronic cases, referral to a mental health professional is called for.

The most important ingredient, however, is the patient. The old joke, "How many psychologists does it take to change a light bulb? One. But the light bulb has to want to change!" applies here. The patient has the ultimate power to make the decision to get better and to manage the disease instead of letting the disease manage him or her. I believe that is the definition of free will. We are the highest level of animals on the planet because we possess free will.

Free will doesn't mean choosing vanilla over chocolate, or having the freedom to eat as many French fries as one is capable of ingesting in a lifetime. It is the freedom to identify when there is an intellectual-emotional mismatch getting in your way and to make the decision to change it. It is the courage to look under the radar at what obstacles are blocking you from achieving your personal goals and succeeding. This journey cannot be accomplished alone, and there is a great support system out there beginning with your cardiologist, to whom you have already entrusted your life. I can assure you that there will be hurdles along the way, but remember that perfection is not a human quality. The important thing is to keep trying, and to make the journey of good mental and physical health a life-long process that will undoubtedly provide satisfaction, wisdom, and contentment, if taken seriously. In addition, the ripple effect of one's success and gains in personal strength along the way will a have profound effect on relationships with family, friends, and business associates. We are all programmed with the necessary software to achieve greatness. The name of that software is "free will," and there is no better way to exercise it than to choose to be healthy and wise.

9. The Body's Perfect Storm

This is the chapter where the healing begins, so pay attention. Rather than focus on what things you need to do right, let's focus on many different lifestyle characteristics that statistically increase your likelihood of having a heart attack when present. If I were the chef of coronary artery disease, what would be my favorite recipe? How would I build the perfect heart attack? Perhaps if you are currently following this recipe, you will now begin to deeply understand why you are doing it and why you need to stop. I will exclude non-modifiable cardiac risk factors, such as age, sex, and family history of coronary disease, because you have no control over these characteristics.

I would start with a middle-aged or older adult and make such a person a smoker with a full-time job that requires way more pounds of flesh than the paycheck looks like on Friday. I would make the job seem so onerous that the person perceives no time to exercise, relax, or do anything just for himself or herself. The person would likely come from a household with two working adults in which costs of living are high and just about equal to or slightly greater than the extent the budget can stretch. Time is a difficult commodity, and many meals are prepared by a frozen food corporation, super market, deli, or fast food chain. Breakfasts are often bread or sweet-based foods, such as bagels, toast, doughnuts, sugar-based cereals, and the like. Lunches are often fast takeout of some sort, and dinners may consist of delivered pizza, large portions of pasta, potatoes, or bread. My recipe patient would be either overweight for his height, or frankly obese, predominantly in the abdominal section.

As a result of this lifestyle and overweight status, he or she is most often hypertensive, and now more and more is turning diabetic. Then, let the above combination, or many permutations thereof, simmer for a decade or two, or three. If nothing is done to change that stew, there is only one possible result…coronary artery disease and myocardial infarction.

Let's apply the principles we have learned from this book to the all-too-common scenario described in our recipe patient. A most important ingredient that permeates the background of our recipe is chronic stress, in the form of either psychosocial stress or emotional difficulties such as depression and anxiety disorders. Our patient has a thirty year mortgage amount of stress, has very little job latitude, likely has marital stress from the severe time constraints, and has dedicated very little time to activities that are either socially engaging or promoting of a support structure. Our patient has slowly cut himself or herself off by being too busy.

This level of stress and difficulty with time management results in convenient food choices with nutrition likely last on the list for consideration. We are a country that eats foods with a high glycemic index, which you now understand leads to weight gain, which leads to high blood pressure and diabetes. But that's not all. The least talked-about and possibly most important factor that changes physically to cause heart disease is the chronic elevation of cortisol levels that occurs in the presence of chronic stress. This hormone, initially designed to provide the bloodstream with glucose for energy when running away from a predator, remains constantly elevated during chronic stress because the body keeps interpreting the outside environment as stressful. This results in a chronic craving for carbohydrates by the individual, because carbohydrates are the source of the glucose that the cortisol is trying to provide for the perceived "needed" energy. The carbohydrate craving thus helps to further fuel the cycle of poor dietary choices, weight gain, and all that follows.

In the metabolic syndrome, which status our patient has now achieved by virtue of abdominal obesity, hypertension, and diabetes, there are common lipid abnormalities that further lead to atherosclerotic plaque formation and coronary artery disease. In this population of patients, high triglycerides and low HDL cholesterol are quite prevalent. To this point, we have trashed many carbohydrates, but we haven't even talked about saturated (animal) fat. In retrospect, we might have added some characteristics to our recipe patient such as being a beef- and dairy-loving individual. In this way we could make an argument that his or her total cholesterol and LDL cholesterol levels would be elevated as well—both potent cardiac risk factors.

Now simmer. A plaque that grows in a coronary vessel takes time. The hypertension constantly provides a shearing stress across it that micro-fractures the outer fibrous cap multiple times per day, setting in motion an inflammatory response of healing and growing. Abnormal fats deposit themselves under the cap to form a cholesterol core that has the consistency of toothpaste at body temperature. One day, when the plaque has simmered enough and is ripe, things will drastically change.

Perhaps a puff on a cigarette will take in just enough nicotine or a fit of anger or depression will result in just enough adrenaline being produced such that the blood pressure and heart rate rise very quickly. The rapid rise of these factors shears off the top of the plaque, like the wind ripping off a corrugated roof in a hurricane. Once the inner cholesterol core is exposed to the bloodstream, the body thinks there is a hole in the blood vessel and incorrectly begins to try to make a clot and a scab to plug up the irregular opening in the vessel wall. The clotting cascade is set into motion, and because the vessel was occluded by the plaque fifty percent or more in the first place, it doesn't take much clot formation to jam the rest of the artery and completely occlude blood flow, causing a heart attack.

Thus goes the recipe for the body's perfect storm. If there are themes in common between you and our recipe patient, you need to recognize that, perhaps without realizing it, you have been participating in lifestyle behaviors that are a recipe for disaster. The good news is that such an outcome can be avoided with careful attention, honesty, and some hard work. Learning how to set boundaries is a key step toward becoming more proactive about your time and how you want to live your life. You are not being selfish by acknowledging the fact that you need time for yourself regularly, such as an hour three times per week for a hobby or exercise. You owe it to yourself not to sabotage this very valuable time you need for yourself. Once you begin to set boundaries, you can turn to every facet of your life, such as food choices, time at work, time for yourself, and time with your significant other, and alter them to your advantage. As you reflect on your life and where it is today, determine to what extent it shares common ground with our recipe patient, and begin to understand that you can't continue this way or else something's going to give.

10. Where Do I Start?

Chances are, if you have read up to this point, you have a healthy side to you and you want to get right into exercising your free will. Many of the suggestions here have meaning to you, but the idea of "peeling off the layers of your personal onion skin" is daunting and intimidating. You may be asking, "What do I need to know about the field of psychology as it pertains to me, and how do I use it to my best advantage?" A good overview of the various kinds of mental health professionals that are out there is useful, as are the different types of therapy that may be offered. Some therapeutic methods are more amenable than others with regard to their ability to influence a specific emotional deficit.

There are many different types of mental health providers. Some can prescribe medications, and some cannot. Some have different or more extensive training than others. In addition, states vary widely with regard to licensing requirements and requirements for training and skills. Finally, we are living in a day when health insurance companies have an increasingly larger say with respect to whom we may or may not choose to see as our health care provider. These are all factors that may come into play when selecting a mental health care provider.

"Psychotherapist" is a broad term for any mental health care provider. This may be a psychiatrist, psychologist, social worker, nurse, marriage and family therapist, or pastoral counselor. Some practitioners set up practices under the heading of "psychotherapist" and have no formal training or aren't subject to any state laws or regulations.

"Psychiatrists" are medical doctors and possess degrees from medical or osteopathic schools. In addition, they have completed at least four years of residency training in psychiatry. They are medical specialists in the diagnosis and treatment of mental illness; they can prescribe medication and can administer psychotherapy. A "board certified" psychiatrist is one who has passed certain exams given by the American Board of Psychiatry and Neurology. I have found that many psychiatrists relegate psychotherapy to psychologists and limit the vast majority of what they do to the medical management of the patient's emotional disorder. While the symptoms of many of the psychological abnormalities discussed in this book can be improved with medication, I feel strongly that a psychotherapy-based approach is the most helpful in order to ensure the best long-term outcome with regard to patient's reactivity and personalization of emotions.

"Psychologists" specialize in psychology: the study of the mind, mental processes, and behaviors. Most often they have a doctoral degree (Ph.D. or Psy.D.). Sometimes therapists with a master's degree in psychology will use the title "psychologist" as well. Generally, psychologists cannot prescribe medication, with certain exceptions in the states of Louisiana and New Mexico. Psychoanalysts are those psychotherapists who are trained to administer a specific type of therapy called psychoanalysis. This method was developed by Sigmund Freud and explores the unconscious and its relationship to factors that influence current interpersonal relationships and behaviors. While "psychoanalyst" is not a legal term, it usually denotes having had extensive training or certification, often in a psychoanalytic institute. The training includes at least four years of psychoanalytic training, coursework, performed supervised psychoanalysis of patients, and undergoing individual psychoanalysis. While individual psychotherapy with a psychologist may vary in its duration, psychoanalysis is more intensive, consisting of multiple sessions per week over a longer duration of time. During a psychoanalysis session, the patient often will lie on a couch without the analyst in sight and speak freely about whatever comes to mind.

"Social worker" is a broad title for professionals trained in helping people with social and health problems. Most have a master's degree and possess the title "M.S.W.," indicating a master's in social work. Training is very variable among social workers, and in order to provide mental health services, they must have advanced mental health training and be licensed in the state in which they are practicing. Licensed clinical social workers (L.C.S.W.) may provide psychotherapy in private practice settings, psychiatric facilities, hospitals, or community facilities. They cannot prescribe medications.

"Psychiatric nurses" are licensed registered nurses (R.N.) who possess additional training in mental health. Their academic degrees may vary from an associate's degree to a bachelor's degree to a master's degree, but it is their level of training and experience that determines what services they can provide. Under a doctor's supervision, they may perform mental health assessments, give psychotherapy, and help patients manage their medications. An advanced practice registered nurse (A.P.R.N.) has at least a master's degree in psychiatric-mental health nursing. Specifically, these nurses may diagnose and treat mental illness. In many states they are licensed to prescribe medications and may practice independently with a physician's supervision.

"Mental health counselors" provide psychological counseling. Most have at least a master's degree in social work or a related field. They have several years of supervised work experience and are licensed or certified. Mental health counselors are capable of offering help in problems ranging from anxiety to depression, job stress to grief. They may also specialize in specific areas such as substance abuse or marriage issues. These counselors may work in a private practice setting or become affiliated with hospitals or community agencies.

"Marriage and family therapists" generally treat disorders within the context of the family. Their therapy is often problem-oriented and solution-based. Although the majority have a master's or doctoral degree, not all states require licensing and certification.

Pastoral counselors are trained mental health providers who also have extensive religious or theological training. They provide psychotherapy and emotional support in a spiritual context.

*

"Psychotherapy" refers to the particular way of treating mental and emotional disorders by way of talking to a mental health professional. Goals of psychotherapy include: learning about the causes of your condition so you can better understand it, learning how to identify and change behaviors or thoughts that adversely affect your life, exploring relationships and experiences, finding better ways to cope with and solve problems, and learning to set realistic goals for your life. Psychotherapy is helpful in alleviating symptoms of emotional distress, and it helps patients gain a sense of contentment and control over their lives. The following is a description of some of the forms of psychotherapy that exist. While it is not an exhaustive list, it introduces the essential methods I have witnessed that have helped many of my cardiac patients.

"Behavior therapy" is aimed at changing unwanted or unhealthy behaviors. It employs a system of rewards or positive reinforcements for appropriate behavior. Often, it involves the utilization of a process called "desensitization," which involves confronting those things that cause anxiety.

I attend to a morbidly obese seventy-three-year-old male who is eleven years post bypass surgery. He is diabetic and has high cholesterol, hypertension, and obstructive sleep apnea. He has obsessive-compulsive behavior, as evidenced by his frequent checking and re-checking of his kitchen pantry to see if he has enough food in the house. It is necessary for him to drive quite a distance to see me in the office, and on one occasion he confessed to me that he plans his journeys by determining which delicatessen he can stop at either on the way to the office or on the way home. His favorite choice on the menu was an egg salad sandwich on white bread with extra mayonnaise.

One way we combated his unhealthy habit was to begin to schedule appointments in the late afternoon, sufficiently later than lunchtime, and ensure that he ate a "reasonable" lunch prior to coming to see me. We talked about his issue of feeling that food was such a necessary provider of security and something he could control, and we made a few fairly closely scheduled visits for him to confront the commute to and from my office without succumbing to his impulsive overeating. This has been fairly effective for this patient and remains in effect to this day. This example of desensitization helped the patient put an end to his unwanted behavior of turning a doctor appointment into a high-fat, high-calorie excursion.

*

"Cognitive therapy" attempts to help the patient identify and change distorted thought (cognitive) patterns that have led to feelings and behaviors that are troublesome, self-defeating, or self-destructive. It is based on the idea that our feelings and behaviors are determined by how we interpret our experiences in life. As with behavior therapy, cognitive therapy focuses on the current problem and does not delve into past issues or conflicts. As opposed to behavior therapy, experiences are the important aspect of the cognitive therapy process.

Cognitive therapy brings to mind a fifty-four-year-old man I take care of. He had an MI about two years ago and is being treated for hypertension and hyperlipidemia (elevated cholesterol). He came into the office for a "sick" visit because of poorly controlled blood pressure readings he had observed over the previous two weeks. Upon questioning, I found out that he was having problems with a tenant in a building that he owned. The tenant owed him 450 dollars and was moving out. What was most upsetting to him was that his wife, while trying to be protective of her husband's medical problems, was taking the position that the 450 dollars were not worth getting high blood pressure over and was willing to forget the whole thing. This made my patient very angry, and according to him, this was the actual cause of the breakthrough high blood pressure.

The patient illustrated here was stuck on needing to be right about the finances with the tenant, and his whole point was not to be cheated out of money that was rightfully his. He was very hurt by the tenant's behavior and personalized the entire scenario. Regardless of his blood pressure, he needed his wife to focus on his "correct" position and appear more confrontational. By possessing the behavior of "needing to be right" and having so much anger to go along with it, the patient's blood pressure skyrocketed and pre-disposed him to a potential health catastrophe. While he was correct about being owed the 450 dollars, we decided to work together to diminish his extreme reactivity and to learn how to accomplish things in a healthier manner. For him, this would include learning how not to take it so personally when unfair things happened and how to stick up for his rights in a calmer, more positive, and more confident fashion. By focusing on the current problem and learning from the patient's experience, we were able to synthesize a tool or solution for him to use the next time he felt his emotions were going way up on the reactivity scale.

*

"Cognitive-behavior therapy" tries to combine aspects of both cognitive and behavior therapies. It focuses on identifying unhealthy, negative beliefs and replacing them with healthy, positive ones. It teaches patients that they don't have to be victims of their environments. It works on the belief that your own thoughts, not those of others, determine how you behave. Cognitive-behavior therapy is very useful in the arena of learning about how patients react to their environments and subsequently learning how to acquire the tools necessary for them to become less reactive.

Cognitive-behavior therapy worked well with a sixty-two-year-old female I take care of. She sees me for cardiac prevention and is being treated for hypertension and hyperlipidemia. For years she has experienced severe stress at work. She has been employed as an office manager in an internist's office for many years, and she had risen too high on the salary scale to simply leave the job when the stress level became unbearable. She was very reactive to the doctor's spouse, who worked in the office as well. My patient continually felt as though she was being treated in a condescending fashion, and was so reactive to the heightened emotions surrounding her interactions with this particular co-worker that she developed hypertension that was very difficult to control.

While instituting anti-hypertensive therapy, we were able to maintain a dialogue regarding how she personalizes what goes on in her office and exactly what her perceptions are. Over time, she became able to identify why "her buttons always felt pressed" and even to begin to predict when the "button pressing" was coming. This enabled her to circumvent the stressful feelings and to diminish the stress response in her body. It had a profound effect on her outlook at work and has enabled her to feel successful and strong while performing her job. Once she began to understand why she reacted the way that she did, she began to predict when those feelings would surface and learned how to avoid letting her emotions become full-blown. Upon becoming successful at this "psychological prescription," she developed improved self-confidence and contentment. There is no doubt that her psychological growth has led to improved physical health, as her blood pressure has become much easier to manage.

*

"Art therapy" is based on the premise that creative activities help people get in touch with their feelings. Many of these patients would otherwise have difficulty expressing themselves. This type of therapy can increase self-awareness and improve coping with traumatic experiences. It fosters an overall positive change in the individual. Music, dance, art, and poetry writing are common forms of art therapy.

Much was accomplished for one of my patients by utilizing art therapy. She is a seventy-four-year old with coronary artery disease, has had multiple coronary stents placed, and continued to display obesity, diabetes, high cholesterol and hypertension. She was abused as a child and suffered a lifetime of low self-esteem. It was very difficult for her to access her deep feelings and confront them. However, she was an award-winning sculptor and painter. This sustained her, and throughout her adulthood it allowed her to learn about who she really was inside and how to be comfortable with that person. It provided an outlet for her to come into close contact with her emotions. Her scratching the surface with art therapy eventually led to her finding a talented therapist with whom she was able to accomplish more than she could have ever imagined in the way of gaining personal confidence and strength.

*

"Exposure therapy" is a specific form of behavior therapy that forces exposure to the offending situation. It is sometimes helpful in post traumatic stress disorder. By inducing the anxiety through returning to the event, the patient can develop coping strategies to avoid the same degree of reactivity in the future.

This brings to mind an eighty-two-year-old female patient. We met approximately eleven years earlier when I was called to the emergency room to care for her husband, who was in full cardiac shock. I took him to the cardiac catheterization lab that night, and he was eventually operated on. He survived for approximately seven more years, finally succumbing to prostate cancer.

By now, my old acquaintance had gone on to develop valvular heart disease, was severely hypertensive, and had an abnormally high cholesterol level. Although she would only agree to seek medical attention with me, she was very apprehensive about coming to my office for fear it would reactivate her memories of past visits with her husband and set off an emotional cascade. Her son reached out to me and told me his mom was in need of medical care. After she and I chatted on the phone for quite a while, she finally agreed to come into the office just to talk about her grief and break the ice with regard to examining her feelings about returning to my office. This was quite helpful for her, and now she maintains her appointments without a glitch in order to get the attention she requires.

In this case, sudden exposure to a stimulus that represented prior trauma or an emotionally painful experience allowed the patient to get in touch with her feelings, express them, and learn how to cope with them in order to get the proper health care she needed.

＊

"Interpersonal therapy" is directed at relationships with other people and how to improve one's interpersonal skills. Patients learn how to analyze their interactions with others and how to develop strategies to counteract difficulties in relationships. Very often after a trauma, emotions are reactive and interpersonal relationships may take the brunt of the outbursts. This type of therapy helps decipher where the "traps" in the relationship are and discusses specific solutions for when those recurring problems arise.

A fifty-eight-year-old woman initially came to me for a heart murmur approximately two years ago. She had a history of thyroid cancer, complained of palpitations, and was overweight. An echocardiogram showed a relatively rare, benign tumor in her heart called an atrial myxoma. She required surgery for its removal, and did well. She continued to complain of palpitations over the last year, and she recently came in appearing quite anxious.

She confessed that she was very hostile and angry at home and couldn't control her emotions. It was affecting how she and her husband were relating and had become a significant problem for the two of them. On further history, it turned out that she had been a rape victim at the hands of her stepfather back to when she was a young woman. Approximately two weeks prior to our visit she had gotten word that the stepfather had passed away. This had stirred up many emotions in her, including guilt, anger, sadness, and betrayal. She had begun to react toward her husband with the anger and hurt she really wanted to express to her stepfather. Upon realizing where the magnitude of her anger came from, we were able to work on understanding that her husband had done nothing specifically to warrant that level of emotional reactivity. This has helped her devise strategies to deal with her anger in a healthier manner and has released the "pressure valve" in the household. It is an illustration of using interpersonal therapy to isolate the problem between my patient and her husband and focus on its specific solution.

*

"Psychoanalysis" and "psychodynamic psychotherapy" are both based on the theories of Sigmund Freud. They examine past events and the unconscious mind to better understand what makes you think, feel, and behave the way you do. Psychoanalysis is more intense, with multiple sessions per week. The patient lies on a couch and has no eye contact with the psychologist, who sits behind the patient. Psychodynamic psychotherapy is based on similar theories, but it is less intensive and the patient is face-to-face with the therapist.

These therapies are designed to truly help one gain long-term change. The patient has the opportunity to define those situations in his or her life that continually cause significant emotional reactivity. By delving into past experiences where those emotions first surfaced, patients can understand where, for example, their anger comes from, and stop directing it where it doesn't belong. By dealing with those emotions that have been pushed down under the radar for many years, sometimes decades, the patient can change his or her level of reactivity in current relationships and become much stronger emotionally.

It is important to bear in mind that many aspects of the various types of psychotherapy overlap, and often multiple strategies may be employed in order to gain the optimal therapeutic result. This is merely an introduction for the reader to explain how therapeutic strategies work and what can be expected if this is your first time seeking help. Many strategies, especially during crises, are solution based, saving the psychoanalytic and psychodynamic models for when the "smoke clears" and you can finally begin to work on yourself.

The decision to embark on a course of psychotherapy is an important one. The only examples we get in life are our mother and father. No one hands us a manual on parenting or relationships. There is always something you can learn if you are honest with yourself and strive to be healthy. As you progress and grow throughout therapy, there will surely be periods of pain and difficulty. Everyone experiences this, but those who want greatness for themselves have the staying power to work through the tough times. If you feel an aversion to continuing therapy or are avoiding something painful, chances are there is a conflict going on inside you, and this conflict then becomes the most important topic for you to go into your next session with. Remember, you wouldn't get off the table halfway through your bypass operation, so don't let your therapy be any different!

11. Give Yourself a High Five

It is important for patients to be able to approach their health in a multi-factoral way that is tangible and practical yet comprehensive. While most self-help books are effective in patient education, it is hard for patients to combine information they gather from nutritional books with those addressing exercise, relaxation techniques, smoking cessation, and mental health issues. I believe my five-step guide is useful in that it addresses the five areas patients have the most trouble integrating. If nothing else, it is a great starting point. While these suggestions are not comprehensive, they are extremely practical; they work, and they will get you going in a positive direction by integrating five extremely important topics.

*

Diet is tip number one. As I have observed with many of my patients, nutrition is a difficult subject and one that can be extremely confusing. Most Americans know the importance of eating a low fat diet, which essentially involves minimizing animal fats in the form of meat or dairy products. Olive oil should be the staple fat used in the household for salads or sautéing. Low fat milk should be used for coffee and cereal. That being said, I know that when patients are not compliant with a low fat diet or when they produce cholesterol, I am usually successful in lowering total cholesterol and LDL cholesterol with medication, often a statin drug.

These medications are usually well tolerated and have revolutionized our ability to lower elevated cholesterol levels. While this is not an excuse to go out and binge on fats, it makes carbohydrates the nutrient family most challenging to the patient and clinician.

The area most people need help with is knowledge about the carbohydrate world. Most people are amazed at the glycemic index of the foods they are eating, and I believe that information should be placed in the nutritional information box of every food containing carbohydrate. Thus, my first tip is, "Did you think about glycemic index today?" For example, Cheerios cereal has a glycemic index of 74, white potato 93, and a bagel 72. Pumpernickel bread has a glycemic index that is relatively low at 55.

Virtually any diet book has an exhaustive list of the glycemic index of carbohydrates, and this information can be obtained easily by searching "glycemic index" on your computer's web browser. Become familiar with this list. Bring it to the supermarket when you shop. By substituting low glycemic index foods for high glycemic index foods, you are certain to lose weight, avoid or better control diabetes, and feel a whole lot better. If you think the balance in your checkbook is important to know, it pales in comparison to the importance of becoming more aware of the glycemic index of the foods you eat regularly.

*

Exercise is the second tip toward optimal health. However, nobody said you have to train for the Olympics or keep up with the twenty-five year old next to you on the treadmill at the gym. Twenty minutes of exercise three times per week is all that is necessary for cardiovascular conditioning. At first, just begin introducing your body to dedicating this time to exercise on a weekly basis, and keep a diary. I tell patients not to challenge themselves too much at first, otherwise it won't be fun and they won't gain consistency. Take baby steps. Walk leisurely for twenty minutes. Listen to your favorite music. Get comfortable workout clothes and walking shoes that add novelty to the exercise commitment.

Once you are in a new habit of going to the exercise room, you will automatically progress and make your workouts more challenging in a stepwise fashion. Swimming, elliptical machines, bicycles, and rowing are common aerobic activities that are beneficial. Exercise classes are also a way of being part of a group and of getting through a workout without getting bored or discouraged. Small changes have huge benefits over the long run, so keep with it!

*

Relaxation is the third major area. There are many websites with articles and suggestions for improving your level of relaxation in order to de-stress. Just performing simple deep breathing exercises at red lights is a way to diffuse tension while driving. Common stress reducers include going for a walk, playing with pets, watching a comedy, spending time outdoors, getting in a good workout, listening to music, writing in a journal, getting a therapeutic massage, taking a yoga class, or curling up with a good book. Relaxation tapes are also a way to soothe yourself and are widely available. It is important that patients nurture themselves by participating in relaxation activities regularly. It does not render one selfish. It is essential for all of us to devote this time to ourselves, or else the stress we walk around with will have nowhere to go and inevitably will result in many of the adverse consequences discussed in this book.

*

Smoking cessation is the fourth tip people need to do something about. There is no greater intervention that combats heart disease than quitting smoking. In some studies, it has been shown to reduce death rates from heart disease by as much as fifty percent. Medications have become more effective in this arena and can be life-changing. If you smoke, it is imperative that you look at the calendar today and pick a "quit date." Your doctor can help, and there are numerous support groups and hotlines available for your benefit. I have helped numerous patients quit who could have never imagined themselves without a cigarette, and I strongly urge my readers to join their accomplishment.

*

The fifth and final tip is emotional well-being. On a daily basis, patients need to ask themselves if their behavior is contributing to or detracting from their overall health. If it is detracting from it, and they can't stop, they have intellectual-emotional mismatch and need help bridging the gap. Anxiety, chronic stress, or depression may be lurking underneath the radar and expressing itself through maladaptive behaviors. This is a crucial conversation you must have with yourself and, if necessary, your physician.

*

Dr. Brown's High 5

BMI: ☐

DATE: _____

www.nhlbisupport.com/bmi/
healthy: 18-24.9, overweight: 25-29.9, obese: ≥ 30

I. DID I THINK ABOUT GLYCEMIC INDEX TODAY? ☐ *YES* ☐ *NO*

<u>< =54</u>	<u>55-70</u>	<u>> 70</u>
sweet potato (54)	new potato (62)	white potato (93)
beans (48)	honey (58)	white rice (72)
soy beans (18)	raisins (64)	sugar (100)
cherries (22)	pita bread (57)	donut (76)
soy milk (30)	pumpernickel (55)	french baguette (95)
mixed grain bread (48)	*Life* cereal (66)	white bread (78)
Special K cereal (54)		most cold cereals (74)
Yam (51)		mashed white potato (72)
al dente pasta (<55)		bagel (72)

II. AM I EXERCISING FOR 20 MINUTES THREE TIMES PER WEEK?
☐ *YES*   ☐ *NO*

III. IN ADDITION TO EXERCISE, AM I SPENDING REGULAR TIME (15-30 MIN)
WITH YOGA, ART, MUSIC, MASSAGE, RELAXATION TAPES, OR A MEANINGFUL
PROJECT?   ☐ *YES*   ☐ *NO*

AM I DOING DEEP BREATHING EXERCISES (AT RED LIGHTS)?
☐ *YES*   ☐ *NO*

IV. AM I SMOKING?   ☐ *YES*   ☐ *NO*

  IF NO, QUIT DATE: _____

V. MY OVERALL BEHAVIOR AND CHOICES CONSISTENTLY CONTRIBUTE
TOWARD MY GOOD HEALTH, AND DO NOT DETRACT FROM IT?

☐ *YES*   ☐ *NO*

IF NO, DISCUSS THE POSSIBILITY OF UNDERLYING ANXIETY OR DEPRESSION,
OR CHRONIC STRESS AS IMPORTANT CARDIAC RISK FACTORS WITH YOUR
PHYSICIAN.

Note that at the top of the figure is a box for your body mass index (BMI). This is determined by using the table in Figure 2. By looking for your height in inches on the left side and your weight in pounds on the top, you can find a number that represents your body mass index. Healthy BMI's are below 26. By putting your BMI on top of the sheet first, you can determine how much weight you need to lose in order to be a healthier patient. Many people are amazed at what health professionals consider healthy versus what is considered "slim" in our culture. To be most true to yourself, follow the numbers and try to lower your BMI slowly and consistently if it is elevated.

I have condensed my five tips onto one page that functions as a simple checklist. I have included the glycemic index of many foods for the reader to carry as a guide. It can be individualized by adding common staples in your household to the columns of low, intermediate, and high glycemic index foods. This list should become a part of your everyday "things to do" list, and it will lead to weight loss and improved mental and physical health. Reviewing your BMI on a daily basis will hopefully motivate you to stick with the program until your goal is reached. I feel that this five-step checklist is a perfect place for anyone to start the road to personal success. Once these five pillars of health have become a part of your routine, it will be easier to advance your knowledge of nutrition, exercise, relaxation, and awareness of your emotional health. Feel free to send me an email and tell me how you are progressing! Good luck.

BMI	19	20	21	22	23	24	25	26	27	28	29	30	31	32	33	34	35
Height							Weight in Pounds										
4'10"	91	96	100	105	110	115	119	124	129	134	138	143	148	153	158	162	167
4'11"	94	99	104	109	114	119	124	128	133	138	143	148	153	158	163	168	173
5'	97	102	107	112	118	123	128	133	138	143	148	153	158	163	168	174	179
5'1"	100	106	111	116	122	127	132	137	143	148	153	158	164	169	174	180	185
5'2"	104	109	115	120	126	131	136	142	147	153	158	164	169	175	180	186	191
5'3"	107	113	118	124	130	135	141	146	152	158	163	169	175	180	186	191	197
5'4"	110	116	122	128	134	140	145	151	157	163	169	174	180	186	192	197	204
5'5"	114	120	126	132	138	144	150	156	162	168	174	180	186	192	198	204	210
5'6"	118	124	130	136	142	148	155	161	167	173	179	186	192	198	204	210	216
5'7"	121	127	134	140	146	153	159	166	172	178	185	191	198	204	211	217	223
5'8"	125	131	138	144	151	158	164	171	177	184	190	197	203	210	216	223	230
5'9"	128	135	142	149	155	162	169	176	182	189	196	203	209	216	223	230	236
5'10"	132	139	146	153	160	167	174	181	188	195	202	209	216	222	229	236	243
5'11"	136	143	150	157	165	172	179	186	193	200	208	215	222	229	236	243	250
6'	140	147	154	162	169	177	184	191	199	206	213	221	228	235	242	250	258
6'1"	144	151	159	166	174	182	189	197	204	212	219	227	235	242	250	257	265
6'2"	148	155	163	171	179	186	194	202	210	218	225	233	241	249	256	264	272
6'3"	152	160	168	176	184	192	200	208	216	224	232	240	248	256	264	272	279
	Healthy Weight						Overweight					Obese					

12. Final Thoughts

So much is different in our 21st century world than what we can glean from generations past. Despite technological advances, the United States is thirty-eighth on the list of the world's nations with regard to life expectancy. We are an overweight, unhealthy nation with no remission in sight. Technology has had a great effect on our overall societal health.

Since the industrial revolution and the advent of rolling mills to process grains, the marketplace has become permeated with product after product containing enriched white flour. This process takes natural grains, removes the healthy component, the germ seed, and grinds the stalks to make fine white flour. This is necessary because the heat from the milling equipment will make the seed coat become rancid, so it is removed prior to milling. This process essentially eliminates any nutritional value naturally present in the grain. Why do you see labels of white bread stating, "Enriched with vitamins and minerals"? The answer is that all of the nutritional value was removed prior to processing, and therefore these micronutrients must be added in order to give the bread any nutritional value at all! If you peruse the shelves in virtually any grocery store, you will find that it is quite a challenge to find baked products that do not contain this unhealthy ingredient. The persistence of enriched white flour in the marketplace has resulted in the American diet having an inordinately high glycemic index compared to generations past. This results in high blood sugar levels after meals, which cause insulin levels to be elevated constantly. Chronically high insulin levels promote the storage of calories (weight gain), among other things. High glycemic index diets lead to insulin resistance by the above described down-regulation process and ultimately are a major contributor to the development of diabetes. Because of rolling mills, our baked goods have moved away from the stone-ground, whole grain products to the fluffy, soft, "live on the shelf for a long time" products we have now. That may be fine for corporate America, but their business is to sell bread, cookies, etc., not to help you live longer or healthier.

There is currently a craze about fish oil supplements containing the essential "omega-3 and omega-6" fatty acids. What is that all about? These essential oils are called essential fatty acids because animals don't have the necessary enzymes to make them for themselves, so it is essential that they be acquired in the diet. Salmon, well known to be high in omega-3 and omega-6 fatty acids, are so because all day the fish eat algae that contain significant amounts of these substances, and thus the essential fats get incorporated into the flesh of the fish. Thus, when eaten, the salmon will contain these essential oils. Our ancestors weren't dropping dead of heart attacks like we are because cattle and chickens used to range free all the time, and the grasses they ate worked the same way the algae does in the salmon. The omega-3 and omega-6 fatty acids from the grasses were incorporated into the yokes of eggs and the meat of the animals, which were then ingested by humans.

Today, most poultry and cattle are given "feed." Think of the steakhouse that serves "Only the finest corn-fed beef." These are cattle that are not eating grass, so the provisions produced by them are void of the essential fatty acids. Our bodies are thus not given the right building blocks for the synthesis of cells, hormones, and other vital substances. With faulty raw materials come faulty hormones and the like, which promote disease. While we do eat too much saturated fat in this country, we are also suffering from a significant omega-3 fatty acid deficiency, which translates into aberrant lipid profiles and vascular disease. Simply put, if you don't put the right fuel in the pipes, they will clog like those in any other machine. I advocate to my patients that they eat organic dairy and meat products for the simple reason that the animals producing these products have been free-ranging, and thus their provisions are not void of the essential omega-3 and omega-6 fatty acids.

A third major challenge for us today revolves around changes in social mores and societal patterns. We are a society of pleasure seekers. Fun is a high priority here in America. We don't just enjoy a baseball or football game anymore; it extends from the pregame show to the postgame show, and when that's over, there is always twenty-four hour sports coverage available on television, and so forth. We may work hard, but when work is over, it's time to have fun. So, how has that hurt us?

The matter of what pleasure you're after can make all the difference. One way of looking at pleasures is to categorize them. On the surface, there is *material* pleasure. This consists of material items such as money, nice cars, nice clothes, vacations, and the like. It is fun and gives us pleasure when we are in contact with whatever it is we are after. Material pleasure is short-term pleasure. That's why you have to keep repeating it in order to feel the same pleasure. It is not lasting.

The next category moves into the long-term pleasure realm. *Love* is the next rung on the "pleasure ladder." There is no amount of money that can buy it; it is a completely separate entity. Think of the love one has for one's children. Would anyone give up his or her child for a million dollars? I don't think so. Love is a long-term pleasure we cannot live without.

The next rung on the "pleasure" ladder is something that people risk losing relationships for, but it is deeper and is also a long-term pleasure. It is a *cause*. What do you believe in? What is it that people are willing to die for? It is their cause. They will leave loved ones to pursue a cause. This goes on every day in our world. We have young men dying in Iraq and Afghanistan who are fighting for freedom and democracy. They are heroes, and the deep pleasure they achieve by representing their cause can not compare to owning a new flat screen television.

An alternative way of looking at this "pleasure principle" is to consider short-term material pleasure as "bodily" pleasure and long-term pleasure, love and causes, as "soul" pleasure. Our country was formed and based on civic duty, community, and religious affiliation, all of which embody social support and structure, relationships and causes. Modern day culture focuses on the "me", not the "we," and has moved more toward individuality. We sit at computers and televisions. Kids have one-on-one play dates. Video games keep us indoors and away from groups. We are focusing on the lowest level of pleasure instead of creating ways to learn what our purpose is and how to accomplish it. While we need all three types of pleasure to be content, I suggest that, as a whole, the balance in our society has become skewed greatly toward material pleasure, with many people who have great difficulty in relationships and are too locked into their routines to even consider that they may have a cause they could identify their lives with.

After having studied the human race for my entire career, I believe that the changes in the American diet by way of enriched white flour, loss of essential fatty acids from our foods, and alterations in the focus of our society have been perhaps the three most important factors leading to our present-day unhealthy nation.

Previously not well understood in medical and cardiology circles has been the fourth and final component contributing to our poor mental and physical condition. This component is the subject of this book: psychosocial risk factors, which include chronic stressors, depression, and anxiety disorders, including post traumatic stress disorder. While it's easy to say "The stress of my job caused my heart attack," or "He died of a broken heart," it's time to finally recognize that while that may be true, it doesn't stop there. It is my hope that this work has helped define the exact link between emotion and the heart attack and relate the occurrence of the heart attack to the difficult emotions. Without this, we as physicians and patients have no chance to learn about how to treat it and how treatment affects our disease and longevity as a culture.

These chronic disturbances of emotion increase sympathetic nervous system activation and further activate the hypothalamic-pituitary-adrenal axis of hormones, resulting in chronically increased noradrenaline and cortisol levels. Noradrenaline's actions

increase heart rate and blood pressure, render the heart suscep-
tible to myocardial ischemia, and increase the likelihood of a cardiac arrhythmia. Cortisol increases blood sugar levels in order to
help the body deal with stress, but in chronically elevated states,
it leads to the craving of carbohydrate, abdominal obesity, diabetes and the metabolic syndrome.

It is more important than ever that patients and doctors recognize the various psychosocial risk entities so that they may be
addressed properly and thoroughly. Much can be done to improve
nutrition, aid smoking cessation, and control cholesterol and hypertension. In addition, stress management and relaxation techniques need to be introduced to the appropriate patients, and
depression and anxiety disorders must be dealt with accordingly.
Recognition and supportive psychotherapy are an excellent start
for the clinician, saving the more difficult cases for intervention
with medication or referral to a psychologist or psychiatric. The
use of selective serotonin receptor inhibitors have been shown to
be safe for the cardiac population and effective for depression,
anxiety disorders, and post traumatic stress disorder. There is
clearly so much more that we can all do together in the realm of
prevention, above and beyond our compulsive tracking of the traditional cardiac risk factors.

I have also observed one fallacy among patients that gets in
the way frequently. More common in the male population, but
prevalent enough in females, is what I call the "macho" complex.
Many cardiac patients view themselves as the patriarch or matri-
arch of the family and are afraid to confront difficult emotions.
They have a misconception that admitting to feelings of fear or
anxiety will label them as "weak" individuals. They perceive
themselves as the backbones of the family unit and therefore don't
give themselves the latitude to be the ones in need. Common sen-
timents include: "What would they all do without me?" or "I
can't show my weakness." Just as heart disease is not your fault,
neither is emotional difficulty. As you can see, it's part of human
nature. Often when people are overcome with depression, anxiety,
or panic, they further punish themselves for being "weak" or
making life more difficult for everyone else. As a defense mecha-
nism, they try to push all their emotions under the rug and not

to show their colors. You now know this will only work temporarily and is ultimately a recipe for ill health and the worsening of one's clinical condition.

My final thoughts wouldn't be complete without a few words addressing the all-too-common behavior called denial. Denial is an extreme form of avoidance behavior with great potential for tragic consequences. It is usually recognized retrospectively because patients in denial often don't get to medical attention on time. I have seen patients present to the hospital after severe damage has been done, or worse, too late for me to resuscitate them. I implore anyone reading this book to listen to your body. I am amazed by women who drink alcohol or smoke and are able to stop everything when they realize they are pregnant, yet can't empower themselves to give up the same habits purely for their own benefit when they are not pregnant. Nurture yourself as you would your child. Set realistic expectations of how many hours a week you can work, and plan out what you are going to eat at mealtimes. Live within your means. If you don't feel well or are experiencing chest pains, don't self-diagnose, because I have seen many people make the wrong diagnosis and suffer for it. Antacids are *not* a treatment for undiagnosed chest pain.

Your family will not benefit from your being disabled or absent. Make your health the long-term pleasure you are after and consider it your cause. The benefits of this newly realized cause will be the best gift you can give to yourself and your loved ones. There is no correlation between the degree of one's intelligence and extent of one's denial. It is a universal human tendency that unfortunately can kill.

I am hopeful that after reading this book, patients will come to understand that it is extremely important to introduce themselves to their feelings and what it is that they stand for. We are complex beings with complex bodies and complex emotions. Perhaps the first step is to allow yourself to be a human being after all. Since perfection is not a human quality, you certainly can't be faulted for not being perfect! The concepts introduced here should serve as a guide to patients with risk factors for heart disease and as a comfort to those who have already experienced the overt manifestations of the disease. Emotions are not to be denied but rather recognized and nurtured in the proper way. I hope that this book will help give individuals the courage to understand that many operative forces are at work here, and that while the problem is a complicated one, the true solution resides deep within all of us. The recognition, acceptance, and opportunity that our emotions can provide us with are a pathway toward success, not failure. I urge all of my readers to begin the good, hard work necessary to determine what is getting in their way. It is a worthy journey with many benefits above and beyond an improved cholesterol profile on your next blood test. The time has come for all of us to put on our "special glasses" and see firsthand within ourselves that specific, individual cure. It is there if you look hard for it. It is right there, somewhere under the radar.

Acknowledgement

I would like to acknowledge Dr. Alan Rozanski as a mentor, professor, and catalyst for me to write this book. I met Alan when I was a fellow in cardiovascular disease at St. Luke's Hospital, New York. In addition to sharing with me his unparalleled expertise in nuclear cardiology and the detection of coronary artery disease, Alan taught me how to seek wisdom and truth in this world. His never-ending enthusiasm in the arena of teaching fellows, residents, and medical students everything from clinical cardiology to human nature and psychology is contagious and has touched countless lives.

His initial publications linking mental stress to coronary artery disease were groundbreaking and became a major foundation for the emerging field of behavioral cardiology before its time. His ability to see the "big picture" in human nature and the world fascinated me and led to my ability to view my patients in the way this book is fashioned.

He has involved me in his teaching, his research, and his life, and for that I will always be grateful.

Glossary of Acronyms

ACE	Angiotensin converting enzyme
AICD	Automatic implantable cardioverter defibrillator
AIDS	Acquired immunodeficiency syndrome
ARB	Angiotensin receptor blocker
BMI	Body Mass Index
CABG	Coronary artery bypass graft
CAD	Coronary artery disease
CHF	Congestive heart failure
DSM-IV	Diagnostic and Statistical Manual of Mental Disorders, 4th edition
EF	Ejection fraction
EKG	Electrocardiogram
FDA	Food and Drug Administration
HDL	High density lipoprotein
HPA	Hypothalamic pituitary adrenal axis
LDL	Low density lipoprotein
MI	Myocardial infarction
PTSD	Post traumatic stress disorder
SSRI	Selective serotonin reuptake inhibitor
TNF	Tumor necrosis factor

Bibliography

American Psychiatric Association. 2000. *Diagnostic and statistical manual of mental disorders*. 4th ed. revised. Washington: American Psychiatric Association.

Bankier, B., J. L. Januzzi, and A. B. Littman. 2004. The high prevalence of multiple psychiatric disorders in stable outpatients with coronary heart disease. *Psychosom. Med.* 66: 64550.

Barlow, D. H. 2002. *Anxiety and its disorders*. 2d ed. New York: Guilford.

Baum, A., J. P. Garofalo, and A. M. Yali. 1999. Socioeconomic status and chronic stress: Does stress account for SES effects on health? In *Socioeconomic status and health in industrial nations: Social, psychological, and biological pathways*, ed. N. Adler, M. Marmot, B. S. McEwen, and J. Steward, 131–144. Annals of the New York Academy of Sciences, New York.

Beck, A. T., R. A. Steer, and M. A. Garbin. 1988. Psychometric properties of the Beck Depression Inventory: Twenty-five years of evaluation. *Clin. Psychol. Rev.* 8:77–100.

Bennett, P., and S. Brooke. 1999. Intrusive memories, post-traumatic stress disorder and myocardial infarction. *Br. J. Clin. Psychol.* 38:411–6.

Berkman, L. F., L. Leo-Summers, and R. I. Howwitz. 1992. Emotional support and survival after myocardial infarction: A prospective, population-based study of the elderly. *Ann. Intern. Med.* 117:10031009.

Case, R. B., A. J. Moss, N. Case, M. McDermott, S. Eberly. 1992. Living alone after myocardial infarction. *JAMA* 267:515519.

Cohen, S., W. J. Doyle, R. B. Turner, C. M. Alper, and D. P. Skoner. 2001. Emotional style and susceptibility to the common cold. *Psychosom. Med.* 65:652657.

Danner, D. D., D. A. Snowdon, and W. V. Friesen. 2001. Positive emotions in early life and longevity: Findings from the nun study. *J. Pers. Social Psychol.* 80:804813.

Denburg, R., and I. Denburg. 2000. *The diamond diet: A multifaceted path to weight loss, health, and wellness.* Montclair, New Jersey: 4U Bayou.

Doerfler, L. A., and J. A. Paraskos. 2004. Anxiety, posttraumatic stress disorder, and depression in patients with coronary heart disease: A practical review for cardiac rehabilitation professionals. *J. Cardiopulm. Rehab.* 24:414421.

. 2005. Post-traumatic stress disorder in patients with coronary artery disease: Screening and management implications. *Can. J. Cardiol.* 21:689697.

Doerfler, L. A., J.A. Paraskos, and L. Piniarski. 2005. Relationship of quality of life and perceived control with posttraumatic stress disorder symptoms 3 to 6 months after myocardial infarction. *J. Cardiopulm. Rehab.* 25:166172.

Domino, F. J., and N. M. Kaplan. Overview of hypertension in adults. http://www.uptodate.com/.

ENRICHD Investigators. 2001. Enhancing recovery in coronary heart disease (ENRICHD) study intervention: Rationale and design. *Psychosom. Med.* 63:747755.

Foa, E. B., D. S. Riggs, C. V. Dancu, and B. O. Rothbaum. 1993. Reliability and validity of a brief instrument for assessing posttraumatic stress disorder. *J. Traumatic. Stress.* 6:459473.

Foa, E. B., and E. A. Meadows. 1997. Psychosocial treatments for posttraumatic stress disorder: A critical review. *Ann. Rev. Psychol.* 48:449480.

Foa, E. B., L. Cashman, L. Jaycox, and K. Perry. 1997. The validation of a self-report measure of posttraumatic stress disorder: The posttraumatic diagnostic scale. *Psychol Assess.* 9:445451.

Frasure-Smith, N., F. Lesperance, G. Gravel, A. Masson, M. Juneau, M. Talajic, M. G. Bourassa. 2000. Social support, depression, and mortality during the first year after myocardial infarction. *Circulation* 101:19191924.

Gallo, L. C., W. M. Troxel, L. H. Kuller, K. Sutton-Tyrrell, D. Edmundowicz, K. A. Matthews. 2003. Marital status, marital quality, and atherosclerotic burden in postmenopausal women. *Psychosom. Med.* 65:952962.

Glassman, A.H., C. M. O'Connor, R. M. Califf, K. Swedberg, P. Schwartz, J. T. Bigger, Jr., K. R. Krishnan, L. T. van Zyl, J. R. Swenson, M. S. Finkel, C. Landau, P. A. Shapiro, C. J. Pepine, J. Mardekian, W. M. Harrison, D. Barton, M. McIvor; Sertraline Antidepressant Heart Attack Randomized Trial (SADHEART) Group. 2002. Sertraline treatment of major depression in patients with acute MI or unstable angina. *JAMA* 288:701709.

Gorkin, L., E. B. Schron, M. M. Brooks, I. Wiklund, J. Kellen, J. Verter, J. A. Schoenberger, Y. Pawitan, M. Morris, S. Shumaker. 1993. Psychosocial predictors of mortality in the cardiac arrhythmia suppression trial-1 (CAST-1). *Am. J. Cardiol.* 71:263267.

Green, B. L., S. A. Epstein, J. L. Krupnick, J. H. Rowland. 1997. Trauma and medical illness: Assessing trauma-related disorders in medical settings. In *Assessing psychological trauma and PTSD*, ed. J. P. Wilson and T. Keane,160191. New York: Guilford.

Haines, A. P., J. D. Imeson, and T. W. Meade. 1980. Psychoneurotic profiles of smokers and non-smokers. *Br. Med. J.* 280:1422.

Hamner, M., N. Hunt, J. Gee, R. Garrell, R. Monroe. 1999. PTSD and automatic implantable cardioverter defibrillators. *Psychosomatics* 40:8285.

Hare, D. L., and C. R. Davis. 1996. Cardiac depression scale: Validation of a new depression scale for cardiac patients. *J. Psychosom. Res.* 40:379386.

Jackson, E., and I. S. Ockene. Cardiovascular risk of smoking and benefits of smoking cessation. http://www.uptodate.com/.

. Obesity, weight reduction, and cardiovascular disease. http://www.uptodate.com/.

Januzzi, J. L., T. A. Stern, R. C. Pasternak, and R. W. DeSanctis. 2000. The influence of anxiety and depression on outcomes of patients with coronary artery disease. *Arch. Intern. Med.* 160:19131921.

Joos, S. K., and D. H. Hickam. 1990. How health professionals influence health behavior: Patient provider interaction and health care outcomes. In *Health behavior and health education: Theory, research, and practice*, ed. K. Glanz, F. M. Lewis, and B. K. Rimer, 216241. San Francisco, California: Jossey-Bass.

Karasek, R., D. Baker, F. Marxer, A. Ahlbom, and T. Theorell. 1981. Job decision latitude, job demands, and cardiovascular disease: A prospective study of Swedish men. *Am. J. Public Health* 71:694705.

Kawachi, I., D. Sparrow, P. S. Vokonas, and S. T. Weiss. 1994. Symptoms of anxiety and risk of coronary heart disease: The normative aging study. *Circulation* 90:22252229.

Kawachi, I., G. A. Colditz, A. Ascherio, E. B. Rimm, E. Giovannucci, M. J. Stampfer, W. C. Willett. 1994. Prospective study of phobic anxiety and risk of coronary heart disease in men. *Circulation* 89:19921997.

Kubzansky, L.D., D. Sparrow, P. Vokonas, and I. Kawachi. 2001. Is the glass half empty or half full? A prospective study of optimism and coronary heart disease in the normative aging study. *Psychosom. Med.* 63:910916.

Kutz, I., H. Shabtai, Z. Solomon, M. Neumann, and D. David. 1994. Post-traumatic stress disorder in myocardial infarction patients: Prevalence study. *Isr. J. Psychiatry Relat. Sci.* 31:4856.

Marmot, M.G., H. Bosma, H. Hemingway, E. Brunner, and S. Stansfeld. 1997. Contribution of job control and other